MRI
at a Glance

This new edition is also available as an e-book.
For more details, please see
www.wiley.com/buy/9781119053552
or scan this QR code:

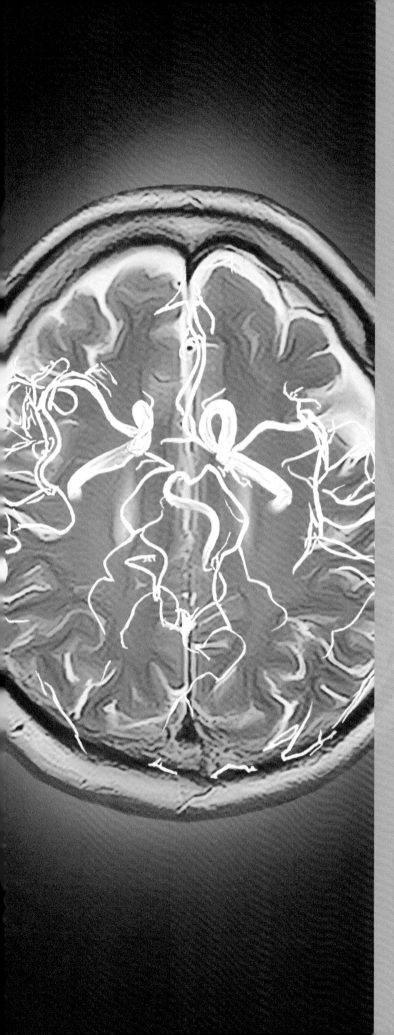

MRI
at a Glance

Third Edition

Catherine Westbrook
Department of Medicine and Healthcare Science
Faculty of Medical Science
Anglia Ruskin University
Cambridge, UK

WILEY Blackwell

Library of Congress Cataloging-in-Publication Data

Westbrook, Catherine.
  MRI at a glance / Catherine Westbrook. — Third edition.
     pages cm
  Includes index.
  ISBN 978-1-119-05355-2 (pbk.)
  1. Magnetic resonance imaging—Outlines, syllabi, etc.   2. Medical physics—Outlines, syllabi, etc.
I. Title.
  RC78.7.N83W4795 2016
  616.07′548—dc23

                                                                    2015022541

A catalogue record for this book is available from the British Library.

Wiley also publishes its books in a variety of electronic formats. Some content that appears in print may not be available in electronic books.

Cover image: © Getty Images/Yuji Sakai

Set in 9.5/11.5pt Minion Pro by Aptara Inc., New Delhi, India

1   2016

Contents

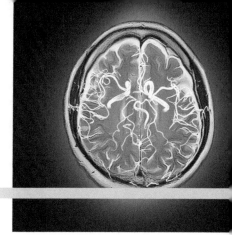

Preface

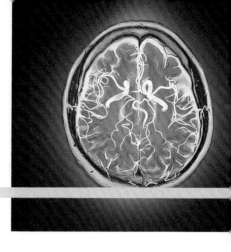

MRI at a Glance is one of a series of books that presents complex information in an easily accessible format. This series has become famous for its concise text and clear diagrams, which are laid out with text on one page and diagrams relating to the text on the opposite page. In this way all the information on a particular topic is summarized so that the reader has the essential points at their fingertips.

The third edition has been updated with a new companion website that includes some exciting new features. In the book, some chapters have been streamlined and reorganized and there are some updated images and diagrams. Each topic is presented on two pages for easy reference and large subjects have been broken down into smaller sections. In the book and companion website I have included simple explanations and animations,

analogies, bulleted lists, simple tables, key points, equations (but only for those who like them), scan tips, 'Did You Know' learning points, some questions and answers and plenty of images to aid the understanding of each topic. There are appendices on trade-offs, acronyms, abbreviations and artefacts. The glossary has also been expanded.

This book is intended to provide a concise overview of essential facts for revision purposes and for those very new to MRI. For more detailed explanations the reader is directed to *MRI in Practice* and *Handbook of MRI Technique*. Indeed, the diagrams and images in this book are taken from these other texts and *MRI at a Glance* is intended to complement them.

Learning MRI physics can be hard work. I hope that this book helps to demystify it!

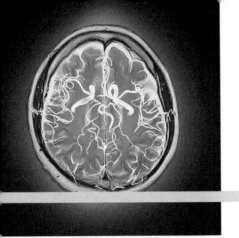

Acknowledgements

Once again I thank my friend and colleague John Talbot for his beautiful diagrams and for his support. We make a great team and long may it continue! Thanks again to Philips Medical Systems and GE for supplying the images, and to all my friends and family in Brighton, London, Paris, Witney, Leeds, St Augustine, Atlanta and New York.

CW

How to use your textbook

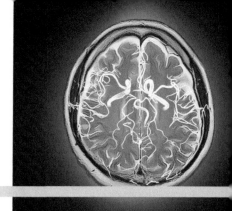

Features contained within your textbook

Each topic is presented in a double-page spread with clear, easy-to-follow diagrams supported by succinct explanatory text.

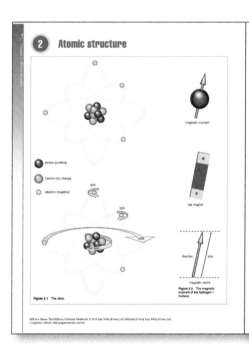

Key point boxes highlight points to remember.

Table 4.3 Key points.

Things to remember:

The magnetic moments of all the spins precess around B_0 at the Larmor frequency that is proportional to B_0 for a given MR active nucleus. Frequency therefore refers to how fast the magnetic moments of spins are precessing and is measured in MHz in MRI.

For field strengths used in clinical imaging, the Larmor frequency of hydrogen is in the radiofrequency band of the electromagnetic spectrum.

Phase refers to the position of a magnetic moment of a spin on its precessional path at any moment in time.

At rest the magnetic moments of the spins are out of phase with each other.

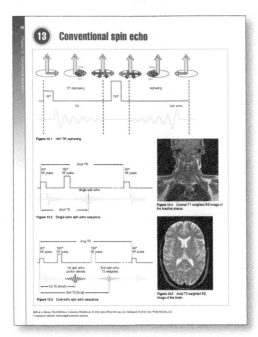

Your textbook is full of photographs, illustrations and tables.

The website icon indicates that you can find accompanying resources on the book's companion website.

About the companion website

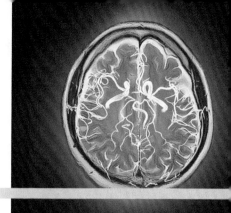

Don't forget to visit the companion website for this book:

www.ataglanceseries.com/mri

There you will find valuable material designed to enhance your learning, including:

- Interactive multiple choice questions
- Animations
- Scan tips, providing useful tips to improve your own MRI technique

Scan this QR code to visit the companion website

MRI Resources from Catherine Westbrook

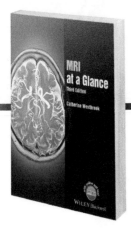
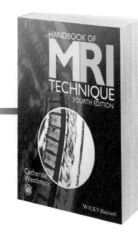
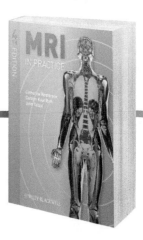

MRI at a Glance, 3rd Edition

- Concisely explains complex information to encapsulates essential MRI physics knowledge
- Includes 55 key points, tables, scan tips, equations, and learning points
- Includes a companion website at www. ataglanceseries.com/mri featuring animations, interactive multiple choice questions, and scan tips to improve own MRI technique
- Ideal for those undertaking the American Registry of Radiation Technologist (ARRT) MRI examination

Publishing January 2016
9781119053552 | 136 pages
£28.99/€38.90/$47.95

Handbook of MRI Technique, 4th Edition

- Guides the uninitiated through scanning techniques and helps the more experienced technologist improve image quality
- Covers theory that relates to scanning and practical tips on gating, equipment use, patient care and safety, and information on contrast media
- Provides step-by-step instruction for examining each anatomical area, with sections on indications, patient positioning, equipment, artefacts and tips on optimizing image quality
- Includes a companion website at **www.wiley.com/go/ westbrook/mritechnique** featuring self-assessment and image flashcards

2014 | 9781118661628 | 392 pages | £42.99/€57.90/$75.900

MRI in Practice, 4th Edition

- Explains in clear terms the theory that underpins magnetic resonance so that the capabilities and operation of MRI systems can be fully appreciated and maximise
- Includes parallel imaging techniques and new sequences such as balanced gradient echo
- Includes a companion website at **www.wiley.com/go/mriinpractice** featuring animated versions of illustrations from the book used on the MRI in Practice Course, and over 200 interactive self- assessment exercises

2011 | 9781444337433 | 456 pages | £36.99/€49.90/$58.99

Catherine Westbrook also offers a range of other educational resources in MRI.

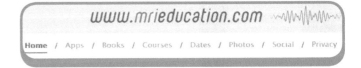

For full details, visit the website at **www.mrieducation.com** where you can find details of the courses and the Apps you can download.

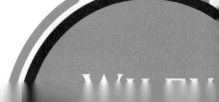

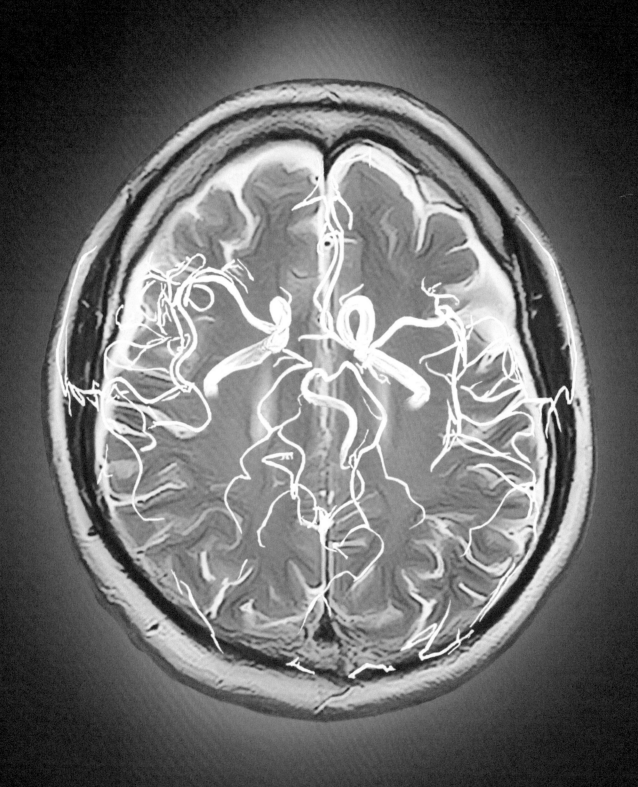

Magnetism and electromagnetism

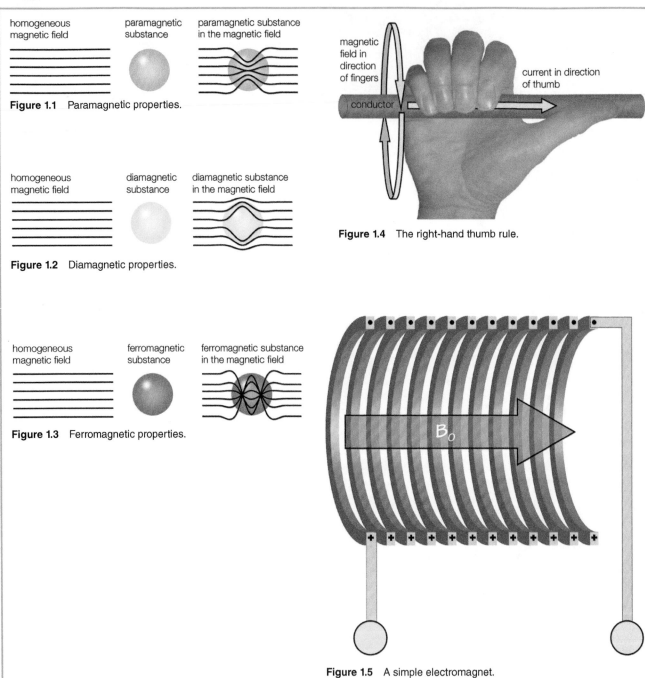

homogeneous
magnetic field

paramagnetic
substance

paramagnetic substance
in the magnetic field

Figure 1.1   Paramagnetic properties.

homogeneous
magnetic field

diamagnetic
substance

diamagnetic substance
in the magnetic field

Figure 1.2   Diamagnetic properties.

homogeneous
magnetic field

ferromagnetic
substance

ferromagnetic substance
in the magnetic field

Figure 1.3   Ferromagnetic properties.

magnetic
field in
direction
of fingers

current in direction
of thumb

conductor

Figure 1.4   The right-hand thumb rule.

B_0

Figure 1.5   A simple electromagnet.

MRI at a Glance, Third Edition. Catherine Westbrook. © 2016 John Wiley & Sons, Ltd. Published 2016 by John Wiley & Sons, Ltd.
Companion website: www.ataglanceseries.com/mri

Magnetic susceptibility

The **magnetic susceptibility** of a substance is the ability of external magnetic fields to affect the nuclei of a particular atom, and is related to the electron configurations of that atom. The nucleus of an atom, which is surrounded by paired electrons, is more protected from, and unaffected by, the external magnetic field than the nucleus of an atom with unpaired electrons. There are three types of magnetic susceptibility: **paramagnetism**, **diamagnetism** and **ferromagnetism**.

Paramagnetism

Paramagnetic substances contain unpaired electrons within the atom that induce a small magnetic field about themselves known as the **magnetic moment**. With no external magnetic field, these magnetic moments occur in a random pattern and cancel each other out. In the presence of an external magnetic field, paramagnetic substances align with the direction of the field and so the magnetic moments add together. Paramagnetic substances affect external magnetic fields in a positive way, resulting in a local increase in the magnetic field (Figure 1.1). An example of a paramagnetic substance is oxygen.

Super-paramagnetism

Super-paramagnetic substances have a positive susceptibility that is greater than that exhibited by paramagnetic substances, but less than that of ferromagnetic materials. Examples of a super-paramagnetic substance are iron oxide contrast agents.

Diamagnetism

With no external magnetic field present, diamagnetic substances show no net magnetic moment, as the electron currents caused by their motions add to zero. When an external magnetic field is applied, diamagnetic substances show a small magnetic moment that opposes the applied field. Substances of this type are therefore slightly repelled by the magnetic field and have negative magnetic susceptibilities (Figure 1.2). Examples of diamagnetic substances include water and inert gasses.

Ferromagnetism

When a ferromagnetic substance comes into contact with a magnetic field, the results are strong attraction and alignment. They retain their magnetization even when the external magnetic field has been removed. Ferromagnetic substances remain magnetic, are permanently magnetized and subsequently become permanent magnets. An example of a ferromagnetic substance is iron.

Magnets are **bipolar** as they have two poles, north and south. The magnetic field exerted by them produces magnetic field lines or lines of force running from the magnetic south to the north poles of the magnet (Figure 1.3). They are called **magnetic lines of flux.** The number of lines per unit area is called the **magnetic flux density**. The strength of the magnetic field, expressed by the notation (**B**) – or, in the case of more than one field, the primary field (**B₀**) and the secondary field (**B₁**) – is measured in one of three units: **gauss (G)**, **kilogauss (kG)** and **tesla (T)**. If two magnets are brought close together, there are forces of attraction and repulsion between them depending on the orientation of their poles relative to each other. Like poles repel and opposite poles attract.

Electromagnetism

A magnetic field is generated by a moving charge (electrical current). The direction of the magnetic field can either be clockwise or counter-clockwise with respect to the direction of flow of the current. **Ampere's law** or **Fleming's right-hand rule** determines the magnitude and direction of the magnetic field due to a current; if you point your right thumb along the direction of the current, then the magnetic field points along the direction of the curled fingers (Figure 1.4).

Just as moving electrical charge generates magnetic fields, changing magnetic fields generate electric currents. When a magnet is moved in and out of a closed circuit, an oscillating current is produced, which ceases the moment the magnet stops moving. Such a current is called an **induced electric current** (Figure 1.5).

Faraday's law of induction explains the phenomenon of an induced current. The change of magnetic flux through a closed circuit induces an **electromotive force (emf)** in the circuit. The emf is defined as the energy available from a unit of charge travelling once around a loop of wire. The emf drives a current in the circuit and is the result of a changing magnetic field inducing an electric field.

The laws of electromagnetic induction (Faraday) state that the induced emf:
- is proportional to the rate of change of magnetic field and the area of the circuit;
- is proportional to the number of turns in a coil of wire Table 1.1);
- is in a direction so that it opposes the change in magnetic field which causes it (**Lenz's law**).

Table 1.1 Common equations of magnetism and electromagnetism.

Equations (if you like them)		
$B_0 = H_0 (1+x)$	B_0 is the magnetic field H_0 is magnetic intensity	This equation shows the apparent magnetization of an atom. A substance is diamagnetic when x < 0. A substance is paramagnetic when x > 0.
$\varepsilon = -Nd\Phi/dt$	ε is the emf N is the number of turns in a coil $d\Phi$ is changing magnetic flux in a single loop dt is changing time	This equation shows that the amount of induced current in a coil is related to the rate of change of magnetic flux (how fast the magnetic lines of flux are crossed) and the number of turns in a coil.

Electromagnetic induction is a basic physical phenomenon of MRI, but is specifically involved in the following:
- the spinning charge of a hydrogen proton causes a magnetic field to be induced around it (see Chapter 2);
- the movement of the **net magnetization vector (NMV)** across the area of a receiver coil induces an electrical charge in the coil (see Chapter 4).

The key points of this chapter are summarized in Table 1.2.

Table 1.2 Key points.

Things to remember:
Paramagnetic substances add to (increase) the applied magnetic field.
Super-paramagnetic substances have a magnetic susceptibility that is greater than paramagnetic substances but less than that of ferromagnetic materials.
Diamagnetic substances slightly oppose (decrease) the applied magnetic field.
Diamagnetic effects appear in all substances. However, in materials that possess both diamagnetic and paramagnetic properties, the positive paramagnetic effect is greater than the negative diamagnetic effect, and so the substance appears paramagnetic.
Ferromagnetic substances are strongly attracted to, and align with, the applied magnetic field. They are permanently magnetized even when the applied field is removed.
Moving a conductor through a magnetic field induces an electrical charge in it.
Moving electrical charge in a conductor induces a magnetic field around it.

2 Atomic structure

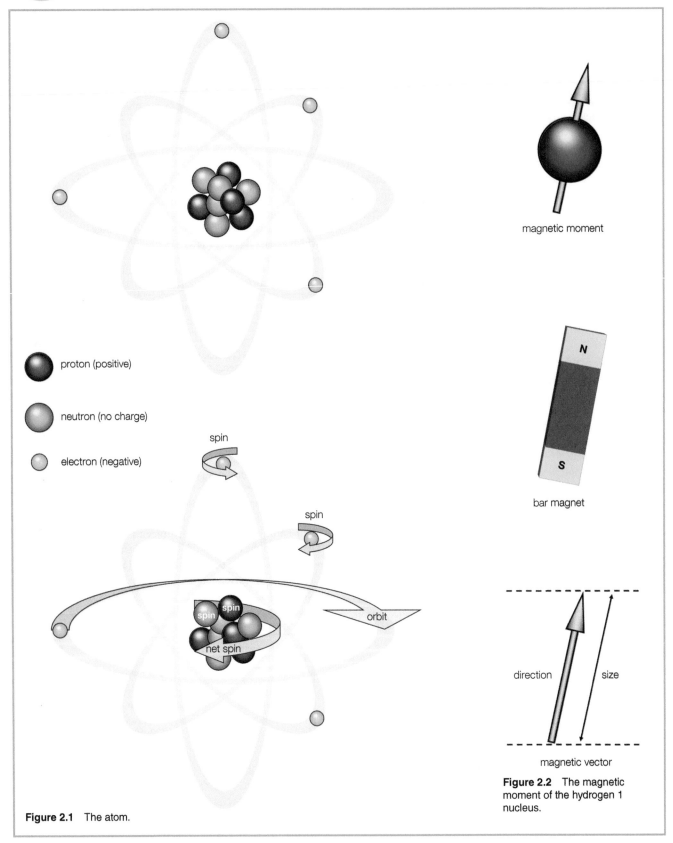

proton (positive)

neutron (no charge)

electron (negative)

spin

spin

spin

spin

net spin

orbit

magnetic moment

N

S

bar magnet

direction   size

magnetic vector

Figure 2.2 The magnetic moment of the hydrogen 1 nucleus.

Figure 2.1 The atom.

MRI at a Glance, Third Edition. Catherine Westbrook. © 2016 John Wiley & Sons, Ltd. Published 2016 by John Wiley & Sons, Ltd.
Companion website: www.ataglanceseries.com/mri

Introduction

Atoms make up all matter in the universe and also therefore in the human body. There are approximately 7 octillion (7×10^{27}) atoms in the average 70 kg person. Most of the human body (96%) is made up of just four elements. These are hydrogen, oxygen, carbon and nitrogen. Hydrogen is the most common element in the universe and in humans.

The atom consists of the following particles:

Protons
- in the nucleus
- are positively charged

Neutrons
- in the nucleus
- have no charge

Electrons
- orbit the nucleus
- are negatively charged (Figure 2.1).

The following terms are used to characterize an atom:
- **Atomic number:** number of protons in the nucleus and determines the type of element the atoms make up.
- **Mass number:** sum of the neutrons and protons in the nucleus.

Atoms of the same element having a different mass number are called **isotopes**. In a stable atom the number of negatively charged electrons equals the number of positively charged protons. Atoms with a deficit or excess number of electrons are called **ions** and the process of removing electrons from the atom is called **ionization.** Only certain types of atoms are available to us in Magnetic Resonance Imaging (MRI). These are atoms whose charged nuclei move or spin. This is because a moving electrical charge produces a magnetic field (see Chapter 1).

Motion within the atom

There are three types of motion of particles in the atom:
- Negatively charged electrons spinning on their own axis.
- Negatively charged electrons orbiting the nucleus.
- Particles within the nucleus spinning on their own axes (Figure 2.1).

Each type of motion produces a magnetic field (see Chapter 1). In MRI we are concerned with the motion of particles within the nucleus and the nucleus itself.

MR active nuclei

Protons and neutrons spin about their own axis within the nucleus. The direction of spin is random, so that some particles spin clockwise and others anticlockwise.

When a nucleus has an *even mass number*, the spins cancel each other out so the nucleus has *no net spin.*

When a nucleus has an *odd mass number,* the spins do not cancel each other out and the *nucleus spins.*

As protons have charge, a nucleus with an odd mass number has a net charge as well as a net spin. Due to the laws of electromagnetic induction (see Chapter 1), a moving unbalanced charge induces a magnetic field around itself. The direction and size of the magnetic field are denoted by a magnetic moment (Figure 2.2). The total magnetic moment of the nucleus is the vector sum of all the magnetic moments of protons in the nucleus. The length of the arrow represents the magnitude of the magnetic moment. The direction of the arrow denotes the direction of alignment of the magnetic moment.

Nuclei with an odd number of protons are said to be **MR active**. They act like tiny bar magnets. There are many types of elements that are MR active. They all have an odd mass number. The common MR active nuclei, together with their mass numbers, are:

hydrogen 1	carbon 13	nitrogen 15
fluorine 19	sodium 23	oxygen 17

The spin characteristics of the commonest MR active nuclei are shown in Table 2.1.

Table 2.1 Constants of selected MR active nuclei.

Element	Protons	Neutrons	Nuclear spin	% Natural abundance
^{1}H (protium)	1	0	1/2	99.985
^{13}C (carbon)	6	7	1/2	1.10
^{15}N (nitrogen)	7	8	1/2	0.366
^{17}O (oxygen)	8	9	5/2	0.038

The isotope of hydrogen called **protium** is the MR active nucleus used in MRI, as it has a mass and atomic number of 1. The nucleus of this isotope consists of a single proton and has no neutrons. It is used for MR imaging because:
- it is abundant in the human body (e.g. in fat and water);
- the solitary proton gives it a relatively large magnetic moment because there are no neutrons present in this type of nucleus. Neutrons tend to decrease the relative size of the nuclear magnetic field, so if they are not present, the magnetic field is maximized (Table 2.1).

In the rest of this book MR active nuclei, and specifically protium, are referred to as *spins*.

The key points of this chapter are summarized in Table 2.2.

Table 2.2 Key points.

Things to remember:

Hydrogen is the most abundant element in the human body.

The nuclei that are available for MRI are those that exhibit a net spin (because their mass number is an odd number).

As all nuclei contain at least one positively charged proton, those that also spin have a magnetic field induced around them (see Chapter 1).

An arrow called a magnetic moment denotes the magnetic field of a nucleus.

 Access the MCQs relating to this chapter on the book's companion website at **www.ataglanceseries.com/mri**

3 Alignment

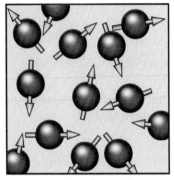
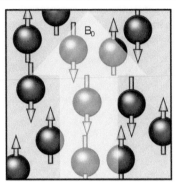

random alignment
no external field

alignment
external magnetic field

Figure 3.1 Alignment: classical theory.

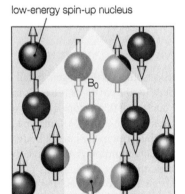
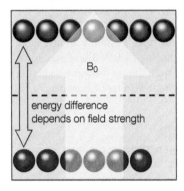

low-energy spin-up nucleus

low-energy spin-up population

high-energy spin-down nucleus

high-energy spin-down population

energy difference
depends on field strength

Figure 3.2 Alignment: quantum theory.

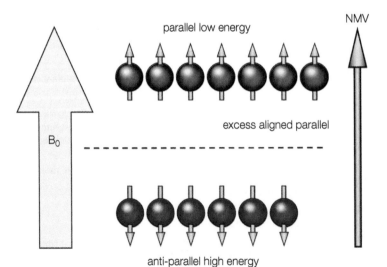

parallel low energy

NMV

excess aligned parallel

anti-parallel high energy

Figure 3.3 The net magnetization vector (NMV).

MRI at a Glance, Third Edition. Catherine Westbrook. © 2016 John Wiley & Sons, Ltd. Published 2016 by John Wiley & Sons, Ltd.
Companion website: www.ataglanceseries.com/mri

In a normal environment the magnetic moments of MR active nuclei (spins) point in a random direction, and produce no overall magnetic effect. When spins are placed in an external magnetic field, their magnetic moments line up with the magnetic field flux lines. This is called **alignment**. Alignment is described using two theories.

The classical theory

This uses the direction of the magnetic moments to illustrate alignment.
- **Parallel alignment**: alignment of magnetic moments in the *same* direction as the main field.
- **Anti-parallel alignment**: alignment of magnetic moments in the *opposite* direction to the main field (Figure 3.1).

At room temperature there are always more spins with their magnetic moments aligned parallel than anti-parallel. The net magnetism of the patient (termed the **net magnetization vector**; **NMV**) is therefore aligned parallel to the main field.

The quantum theory

This uses the energy level of the spins to illustrate alignment. According to the quantum theory, protons of hydrogen nuclei interact with the external magnetic field of the scanner (Zeeman interaction) and cause a discrete number of energy states. For hydrogen nuclei there are only two possible energy states.
- **Spin-up** nuclei have low energy and do not have enough energy to oppose the main field. These are nuclei that align their magnetic moments parallel to the main field in the classical description.
- **Spin-down** nuclei have high energy and have enough energy to oppose the main field. These are nuclei that align their magnetic moments anti-parallel to the main field in the classical description.

The difference in energy between these two states is proportional to the strength of the external magnetic field (B_0). The magnetic moments of the spins actually align at an angle to B_0 due to the force of repulsion between B_0 and the magnetic moments.

What do the quantum and classical theories tell us?

- Hydrogen only has two energy states – high or low. Therefore, the magnetic moments of hydrogen spins only align in the parallel or anti-parallel directions. The magnetic moments of hydrogen spins cannot orientate themselves in any other direction.
- The patient's temperature is an important factor that determines whether a spin is in the high- or low-energy population. In clinical imaging, thermal effects are discounted, as we assume the patient's temperature is the same inside and outside the magnetic field (thermal equilibrium).
- The magnetic moments of hydrogen spins are constantly changing their orientation because they are constantly moving between high- and low-energy states. The spins gain and lose

Table 3.1 Common equations of alignment.

Equations (if you like them)		
$N^+/N^- = e^{-\Delta E/kT}$	N^+ and N^- are the number of spins in the high- and low-energy populations respectively ΔE is the energy difference between the high- and low-energy populations in Joules (J) k is Boltzmann's constant (1.381×10^{-23} J/K) T is the temperature of the tissue in Kelvin (K)	This equation enables prediction of the number of spins in the high- and low-energy populations and how this is dependent on temperature. In MRI, thermal equilibrium is presumed in that there are no significant changes in body temperature in the scan room.

energy and their magnetic moments therefore constantly alter their alignment relative to B_0.
- The number of spins in each energy level can be predicted by the Boltzmann distribution (Table 3.1).
- In thermal equilibrium, at any moment there are a greater proportion of spins with their magnetic moments aligned with the field than against it. This excess aligned with B_0 produces a net magnetic effect called the NMV that aligns with the main magnetic field (Figure 3.3).
- As the magnitude of the external magnetic field increases, more magnetic moments line up in the parallel direction, because the amount of energy the spins must possess to align their magnetic moments in opposition to the stronger field and line up in the anti-parallel direction is increased. As the field strength increases, the low-energy population increases and the high-energy population decreases. As a result, the NMV increases.

The key points of this chapter are summarized in Table 3.2.

Table 3.2 Key points.

Things to remember:
When placed in an external magnetic field, the magnetic moments of hydrogen either align in a spin-up, low-energy or spin-down, high-energy orientation.
At thermal equilibrium, there are more spin-up, low-energy than spin-down, high-energy spins, so the net magnetization of the patient (NMV) is orientated in the same direction as B_0.
The difference in energy between these populations is determined by the strength of B_0.
As B_0 increases the energy difference between the two populations also increases, as the number of spin-up, low-energy spins increases relative to the number of spin-down, high-energy spins.
The signal to noise ratio (SNR) increases at higher values of B_0 (see Chapter 39).

Access the MCQs relating to this chapter on the book's companion website at www.ataglanceseries.com/mri

4 Precession

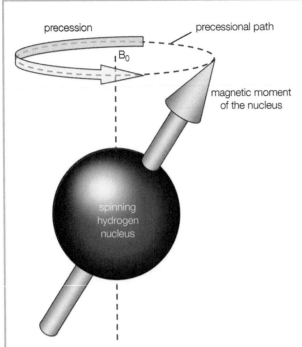

Figure 4.1   Precession.

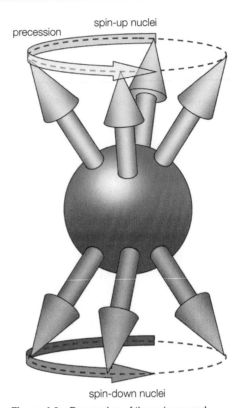

Figure 4.2   Precession of the spin-up and spin-down populations.

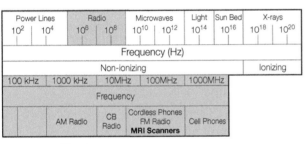

Figure 4.3   The electromagnetic spectrum.

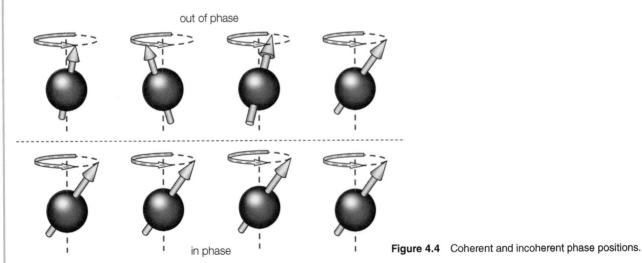

Figure 4.4   Coherent and incoherent phase positions.

MRI at a Glance, Third Edition. Catherine Westbrook. © 2016 John Wiley & Sons, Ltd. Published 2016 by John Wiley & Sons, Ltd.
Companion website: www.ataglanceseries.com/mri

Every MR active nucleus is spinning on its own axis. The magnetic field exerts a torque on the magnetic moments of all MR active nuclei, causing a secondary spin (Figure 4.1). This spin is called **precession** and causes the magnetic moments of all MR active nuclei (spin up and spin down) to describe a circular path around B_0 (Figure 4.2). The speed at which the magnetic moments spin about the external magnetic field is called the **precessional frequency**.

Precessional (Larmor) frequency

The **Larmor equation** is used to calculate the frequency or speed of precession for the magnetic moments of a specific nucleus in a specific magnetic field strength. The Larmor equation is simply stated as follows:

$$\omega_0 = \gamma B_0$$

• The precessional frequency is denoted by ω_0 and expressed in megahertz (MHz).
• The strength of the external field is expressed in tesla (T) and denoted by the symbol B_0 (Table 4.1).
• The **gyromagnetic ratio** is the precessional frequency of the magnetic moments of a specific nucleus at 1T and has units of MHz/T. It is denoted by γ. As it is a constant of proportionality, the precessional frequency or Larmor frequency is proportional to the strength of the external field and can be calculated for any type of MR active nucleus and field strength (Table 4.2).

Table 4.1 Common equations of precession.

Equations (if you like them)		
$\omega_0 = \gamma B_0/2\pi$ *simplified to* $\omega_0 = \gamma B_0$	ω_0 is the precessional of Larmor frequency (MHz) γ is the gyromagnetic ratio (MHz/T) B_0 is the strength of the external magnetic field (T)	This is the Larmor equation. The 2π function enables the conversion of ω_0 from angular to cyclical frequency. As γ is a constant, for a given MR active nucleus ω_0 is proportional to B_0.

Table 4.2 Spin characteristics of selected MR active nuclei.

Element	Nuclear spin	Gyromagnetic ratio (MHz/T)	Larmor frequency at 1.5T (MHz)
^{1}H (protium)	1/2	42.5774	63.8646
^{13}C (carbon)	1/2	10.7084	16.0621
^{15}N (nitrogen)	1/2	4.3173	6.4759
^{17}O (oxygen)	5/2	5.7743	8.6614

The precessional frequencies of the magnetic moments of hydrogen spins (gyromagnetic ratio 42.57 MHz/T) commonly found in clinical MRI are:
• 21.285 MHz at 0.5 T
• 42.57 MHz at 1 T
• 63.86 MHz at 1.5 T (Table 4.2).

The precessional frequency corresponds to the range of frequencies in the electromagnetic spectrum of **radiowaves** (Figure 4.3). Therefore the magnetic moments of hydrogen spins precess at a relatively low radio frequency (RF) compared to other types of electromagnetic radiation. This is why from the perspective of the energies used, MRI is thought to be safe. RF energy is not sufficiently energetic to ionization.

Precessional phase

Phase refers to the position of the magnetic moments of spins on their precessional path at any moment in time. Its units are radians. A magnetic moment travels through 360 radians during one rotation. In this context, frequency is the rate of change phase of magnetic moments; that is, it is a measure of how quickly the phase position of a magnetic moment changes over time. In MRI we are particularly interested in the relative phase position of all the magnetic moments of hydrogen spins in the tissue we are imaging.
• **Out of phase** or **incoherent** means that the magnetic moments of hydrogen spins are at different places on the precessional path at a moment in time.
• **In phase** or **coherent** means that the magnetic moments of hydrogen spins are at the same place on the precessional path at a moment in time (Figure 4.4).

At rest (when the patient is simply placed inside the magnetic field and exposed to B_0), the magnetic moments of the hydrogen spins are out of phase with each other and therefore the NMV does not precess.

The key points of this chapter are summarized in Table 4.3.

Table 4.3 Key points.

Things to remember:
The magnetic moments of all the spins precess around B_0 at the Larmor frequency that is proportional to B_0 for a given MR active nucleus. Frequency therefore refers to how fast the magnetic moments of spins are precessing and is measured in MHz in MRI.
For field strengths used in clinical imaging, the Larmor frequency of hydrogen is in the radiofrequency band of the electromagnetic spectrum.
Phase refers to the position of a magnetic moment of a spin on its precessional path at any moment in time.
At rest the magnetic moments of the spins are out of phase with each other.

Access the MCQs relating to this chapter on the book's companion website at www.ataglanceseries.com/mri

Resonance and signal generation

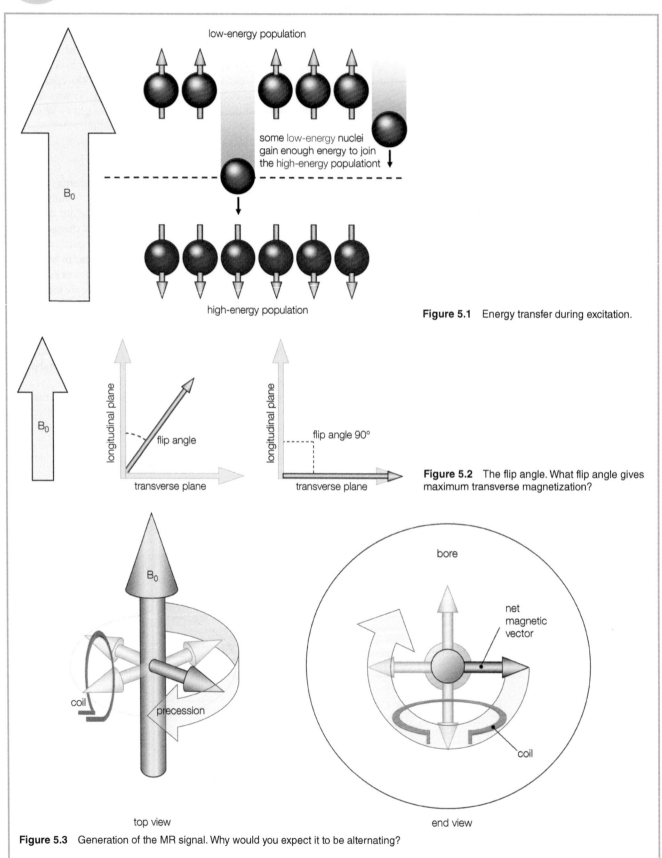

Figure 5.1 Energy transfer during excitation.

Figure 5.2 The flip angle. What flip angle gives maximum transverse magnetization?

Figure 5.3 Generation of the MR signal. Why would you expect it to be alternating?

MRI at a Glance, Third Edition. Catherine Westbrook. © 2016 John Wiley & Sons, Ltd. Published 2016 by John Wiley & Sons, Ltd.

Companion website: www.ataglanceseries.com/mri

Resonance is an energy transition that occurs when an object is subjected to a frequency the same as its own. Resonance is induced by applying a **radiofrequency (RF) pulse**:

- at the same frequency as the precessing magnetic moments hydrogen spins;
- at 90° to B_0.

This causes the hydrogen spins to resonate (receive energy from the RF pulse), whereas other types of MR active nuclei do not resonate. As their gyromagnetic ratios are different from that of hydrogen, their precessional frequencies are also different to that of hydrogen. They only resonate if RF at their specific precessional frequency is applied. As RF is only applied at the same frequency as the precessional frequency of hydrogen, only hydrogen spins resonate. The other types of MR active nuclei do not. Two things happen to the hydrogen spins at resonance: energy absorption and phase coherence.

Energy absorption

The energy and frequency of electromagnetic radiation (including RF) are related to each other and, consequently, the frequency required to cause resonance is related to the difference in energy between the high- and low-energy populations and thus the strength of B_0 (Table 5.1). The spin-up, low-energy hydrogen spins absorb energy from the RF pulse (excitation pulse) and move into the high-energy population. At the same time, the spin-down, high-energy spins give energy away and return to the low-energy state. As there are more low-energy spins, the net effect is of energy absorption. This absorption of applied RF energy at 90° to B_0 causes a net increase in the number of high-energy, spin-down nuclei compared to the pre-resonant state (Figure 5.1).

Table 5.1 Common equations of resonance.

Equations (if you like them)		
$E = h\omega_0$	E is the energy of a photon (Joules, J) h is Planck's constant (6.626×10^{34} J/s) ω_0 is the frequency of an electromagnetic wave (Hz)	Planck's constant relates the energy of a photon of electromagnetic radiation to its frequency. Photons are both particles that possess energy and at the same time behave like waves that have frequency (wave particle duality).
$\Delta E = h\omega_0 = h\gamma B_0$	ΔE is the energy difference between the spin-up and spin-down populations h is Planck's constant (6.626×10^{34} J/s) ω_0 is the precessional or Larmor frequency (MHz) γ is the gyromagnetic ratio (MHz/T).	This equation shows that when the energy of the photon matches the energy difference between the spin-up and spin-down populations, energy absorption occurs. This is proportional to the magnetic field strength B_0.

If just the right amount of energy is applied, the number of nuclei in the spin-up position equals the number in the spin-down position. As a result, the NMV (which represents the balance between spin-up and spin-down nuclei) lies in a plane at 90° to the external field (the **transverse plane**) as the net magnetization

lies between the two energy states. As the NMV has been moved through 90° from B_0, it has a **flip or tip angle** of 90° (Figure 5.2).

Phase coherence

The magnetic moments of the spins move into phase with each other (see Chapter 4). As the magnetic moments of the spins are in phase in both the spin-up and spin-down positions and the spin-up nuclei are in phase with the spin-down nuclei, the net effect is one of precession, so the NMV precesses in the transverse plane at the Larmor frequency.

Did you know?

When a patient is placed in the magnet and is scanned, hydrogen spins do not move. Spins are not flipped onto their sides in the transverse plane and neither are their magnetic moments. Only the magnetic moments of the spins move, aligning either with or against B_0. This is because hydrogen can only have two energy states, high or low (see Chapter 3). It is the NMV that lies in the transverse plane, *not* the magnetic moments, nor the spins themselves.

The MR signal

A receiver coil is situated in the transverse plane. As the NMV rotates around the transverse plane as a result of resonance, it passes across the receiver coil, inducing a voltage in it (see Chapter 1). This voltage is the **MR signal** (Figure 5.3).

After a short period of time the RF pulse is removed. The signal induced in the receiver coil begins to decrease. This is because the in-phase component of the NMV in the transverse plane, which is passing across the receiver coil, begins to decrease as an increasingly higher proportion of spins become out of phase with each other. The amplitude of the voltage induced in the receiver coil therefore decreases. This is called **free induction decay** or **FID**:

- 'free' because of the absence of the RF pulse;
- 'induction decay' because of the decay of the induced signal in the receiver coil.

The key points of this chapter are summarized in Table 5.2.

Table 5.2 Key points.

Things to remember:
The application of RF energy at the Larmor frequency causes a net absorption of energy (excitation) and changes the balance between the number of spins in the low- and high-energy populations.
The orientation of the NMV to B_0 depends on this balance. If there are a similar number of spins in each population, the NMV lies in a plane at 90° to B_0 (transverse plane).
Resonance also causes the magnetic moments of all spins to precess in phase. The result is coherent transverse magnetization that precesses in the transverse plane at the Larmor frequency.
If a receiver coil (conductor) is placed in the transverse plane, the movement of the rotating coherent transverse magnetization causes a voltage to be induced in the coil.
When the RF excitation pulse is removed, the magnetic moments of all spins dephase and produce a FID.

Access the MCQs relating to this chapter on the book's companion website at www.ataglanceseries.com/mri

Access Animations 1.1 and 1.2 relating to this chapter at www.westbrookmriinpractice.com/animations.asp

6 Contrast mechanisms

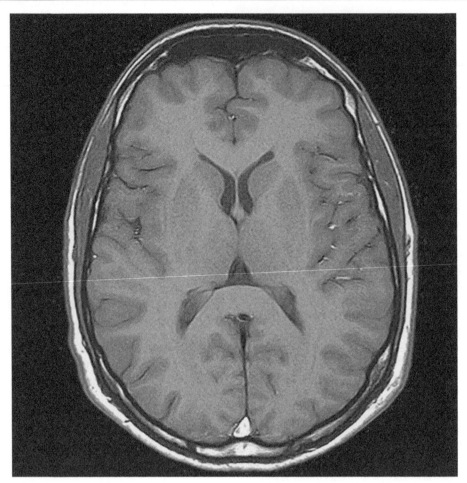

Figure 6.1 An axial image of the brain. Note the difference in contrast between CSF, fat, grey and white matter.

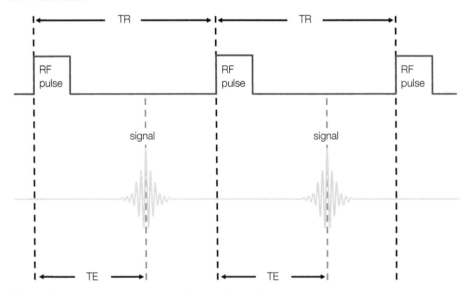

Figure 6.2 A basic pulse sequence showing TR and TE intervals.

MRI at a Glance, Third Edition. Catherine Westbrook. © 2016 John Wiley & Sons, Ltd. Published 2016 by John Wiley & Sons, Ltd.
Companion website: www.ataglanceseries.com/mri

What is contrast?

An image has contrast if there are areas of high signal (white on the image), as well as areas of low signal (dark on the image). Some areas have an intermediate signal (shades of grey, between white and black). The NMV can be separated into the individual vectors of the tissues present in the patient, such as fat, cerebrospinal fluid (CSF), grey matter and white matter (Figure 6.1). The contrast to noise ratio (CNR) is an important image quality parameter (see Chapter 40) and relates to the difference in signal between two adjacent areas. Images demonstrating a good CNR contain large differences in signal intensity. Images demonstrating poor CNR do not.

The determinant of signal intensity in MRI is the magnitude of precessing coherent transverse magnetization that cuts through the windings of the receiver coil when the signal is measured. This is because the amplitude of voltage induced in a conductor depends on the amplitude of the transverse magnetic field (see Chapter 5).

A tissue has a *high signal (white, hyper-intense)* if it has a *large transverse component of magnetization* when the signal is measured. If there is a large component of transverse magnetization, the amplitude of the magnetization that cuts the coil is large, and the signal induced in the coil is also large.

A tissue has a *low signal (black, hypo-intense)* if it has a *small transverse component of magnetization* when the signal is measured. If there is a small component of transverse magnetization, the amplitude of the magnetization that cuts the coil is small, and the signal induced in the coil is also small.

A tissue has an intermediate signal (grey, iso-intense) if it has a medium transverse component of magnetization when the signal is measured.

Image contrast is determined by the difference in signal intensity between tissues. This is controlled by various parameters (Table 6.1).

Table 6.1 Common equations of contrast mechanisms.

Equations (if you like them)		
$SI = PD\, e^{-TE/T2}(1-e^{-TR/T1})$	SI is the signal intensity in a tissue PD is proton density TE is the echo time (ms) T2 is the T2 relaxation time of the tissue (ms) TR is the repetition time (ms) T1 is the T1 relaxation time in the tissue (ms)	This equation shows why the signal intensity from a tissue depends on intrinsic and extrinsic contrast parameters. In gradient echo sequences the flip angle is added to this equation and T2 is referred to as T2* (see Chapter 17).

Extrinsic contrast parameters

These parameters are controlled by the operator. They are:
- **Repetition time (TR)**: This is the time from the application of one RF pulse to the application of the next for a particular slice. It is measured in milliseconds (ms). The TR affects the length of a relaxation period in a particular slice after the application of one RF excitation pulse to the beginning of the next (see Chapter 8 and Figure 6.2).

- **Time to echo (TE)**: This is the time between an RF excitation pulse and the collection of the signal. The TE affects the length of the relaxation period after the removal of an RF excitation pulse and the peak of the signal received in the receiver coil (see Chapter 9). It is also measured in ms (Figure 6.2).
- **Flip angle**: This is the angle through which the NMV is moved as a result of an RF excitation pulse (Figure 5.2).
- **Turbo-factor (TF)** or **echo train length (ETL)** (see Chapter 15).
- **Time from inversion (TI)** (see Chapter 16).
- **'b' value** (see Chapter 25).

Intrinsic contrast mechanisms

These parameters are inherent to the tissue and are not controlled by the operator. They are:
- T1 recovery time (see Chapter 8)
- T2 decay time (see Chapter 9)
- proton density (see Chapter 12)
- flow (see Chapter 46)
- apparent diffusion coefficient (ADC; see Chapter 25)

The composition of fat and water

All substances possess molecules that are constantly in motion. This molecular motion is made up of rotational and transitional movements and is called **Brownian motion**. The faster the molecular motion, the more difficult it is for a substance to release energy to its surroundings.

Fat comprises hydrogen atoms mainly linked to carbon that make up large molecules. The large molecules in fat are closely packed together and have a slow rate of molecular motion due to inertia of the large molecules. They also have a low inherent energy that means they are able to absorb energy efficiently.

Water comprises hydrogen atoms linked to oxygen. It consists of small molecules that are spaced far apart and have a high rate of molecular motion. They have a high inherent energy that means they are not able to absorb energy efficiently.

Because of these differences, tissues that contain fat and water produce different image contrast. This is because there are different **relaxation** rates in each tissue (see Chapters 8 and 9).

The key points of this chapter are summarized in Table 6.2.

Table 6.2 Key points.

Things to remember:
Contrast between tissues occurs because there is a different signal intensity between different tissues.
Signal intensity depends on the amplitude of signal.
Resonance also causes the magnetic moments of all spins to precess in phase. The result is coherent transverse magnetization that precesses in the transverse plane at the Larmor frequency.
If a receiver coil (conductor) is placed in the transverse plane, the movement of the rotating coherent transverse magnetization causes a voltage to be induced in the coil.
When the RF excitation pulse is removed, the magnetic moments of all spins dephase and produce a FID.

Relaxation mechanisms

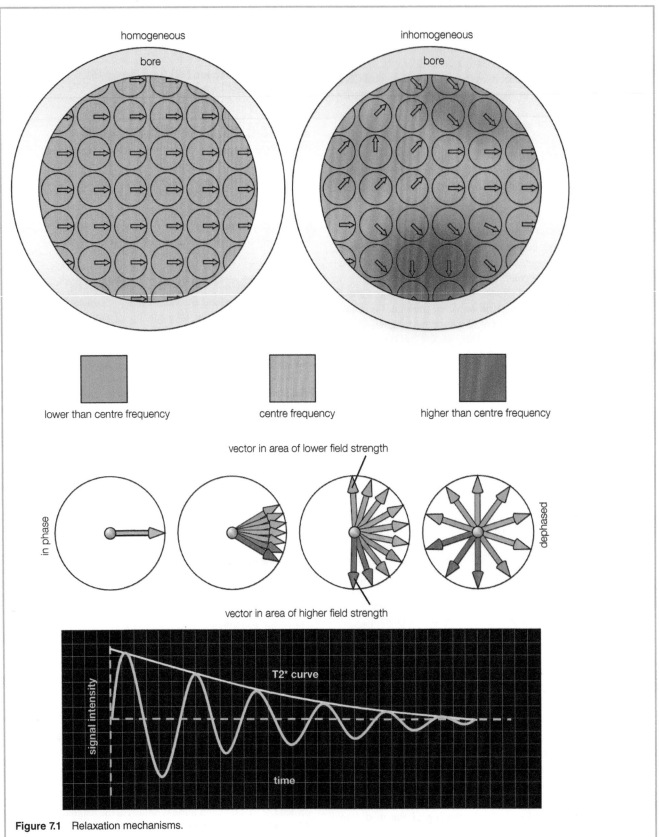

Figure 7.1 Relaxation mechanisms.

MRI at a Glance, Third Edition. Catherine Westbrook. © 2016 John Wiley & Sons, Ltd. Published 2016 by John Wiley & Sons, Ltd.
Companion website: www.ataglanceseries.com/mri

Relaxation is a general term that refers to a loss of energy. In MRI this is energy delivered to the spins via excitation. After the RF excitation pulse has been applied and resonance and the desired flip angle achieved, the RF pulse is removed. The signal induced in the receiver coil begins to decrease. This is because the coherent component of NMV in the transverse plane, which is passing across the receiver coil, begins to gradually decrease as an increasingly higher proportion of spins become out of phase with each other. The amplitude of the voltage induced in the receiver coil therefore gradually decreases. This is called **free induction decay** or **FID**. The NMV in the transverse plane decreases due to:

- relaxation processes;
- field inhomogeneities and susceptibility effects.

The cumulative dephasing of spin-spin interactions and inhomogeneities is called T2* decay (Table 7.1).

Table 7.1 Common equations of relaxation mechanisms.

Equations (if you like them)		
$1/T2^* = 1/T2 + 1/2\,\gamma\Delta B_0$	T2 and T2* are the tissues' T2 and T2* relaxation times (ms) γ is the gyromagnetic ratio (MHz/T) ΔB_0 is the variation in magnetic field (inhomogeneities) (parts per million, ppm)	This equation shows how T2 and T2* are related to each other. Poor field inhomogeneities result in T2* being much shorter than T2, and fast decaying signal.

Relaxation processes

The magnetization in each tissue relaxes at different rates. This is one of the factors that create image contrast.

The withdrawal of the RF produces several effects:
- Spins emit energy absorbed from the RF pulse through a process known as **spin lattice energy transfer** and shift their magnetic moments from the high-energy state to the low-energy state. The NMV recovers and realigns to B_0. This relaxation process is called **T1 recovery**.
- The magnetic moments of the spins lose precessional coherence or dephase and the NMV decays in the transverse plane. The dephasing relaxation process is called **T2 decay**.

The magnetic moments of the spins lose their coherence by:
- interactions of the intrinsic magnetic fields of adjacent nuclei (**spin-spin**) causing **T2 decay** (see Chapter 9);
- **inhomogeneities** of the external magnetic field.

Field inhomogeneities

Despite attempts to make the main magnetic field as uniform as possible via shimming (see Chapter 51), inhomogeneities of the external magnetic field are inevitable and slightly alter the magnitude of B_0; that is, some small areas of the field have a magnetic field strength of slightly more or less than the main field strength.

Due to the Larmor equation, the precessional frequency of the magnetic moment of a spin is proportional to B_0 (see Chapter 4), so spins that pass through inhomogeneities experience a precessional frequency and phase change, and the resulting signal decays exponentially. This results in a change in dephasing of the transverse magnetization due to a loss in phase coherence (Figure 7.1). The resulting signal decays exponentially and is called an FID.

T2 decay is irreversible because spin-spin interactions occur at the atomic or molecular level. However, T2* decay, particularly caused by field inhomogeneity, can be compensated for and is desirable (Table 7.1). In order to produce images where T2 contrast is visualized, ideally there must be a mechanism to rephase spins and compensate for magnetic field inhomogeneities. *Pulse sequences* are mechanisms that perform this function.

A **pulse sequence** is defined as a series of RF pulses, gradient applications and intervening time periods. They enable control of the way in which the system applies RF pulses and gradients. By selecting the intervening time periods, image weighting is controlled. Pulse sequences are required because, without a mechanism of refocusing spins, there is insufficient signal to produce an image. This is because dephasing occurs almost immediately after the RF excitation pulse has been removed.

The main purposes of pulse sequences are to:
- rephase spins and remove inhomogeneity effects and therefore produce a signal or echo that contains information about the T2 decay characteristics of tissue alone;
- enable manipulation of the TE and TR to produce different types of contrast.

Spins are rephased by using (Table 7.2):
- a 180° RF pulse (used in all spin echo sequences);
- a gradient (used in all gradient echo sequences).

Table 7.2 Pulse sequences and their rephasing mechanisms.

Use RF pulses to rephase spins	Use gradients to rephase spins
Conventional spin echo	Coherent gradient echo
Fast or turbo spin echo	Incoherent gradient echo
Inversion recovery	Steady-state free precession
STIR	Balanced gradient echo
FLAIR	EPI

The key points of this chapter are summarized in Table 7.3.

Table 7.3 Key points.

Things to remember:
Relaxation is a general term that refers to a loss of energy. In MRI this is energy delivered to the spins via excitation.
Relaxation and inhomogeneities result in a FID signal.
Spin lattice energy transfer is a relaxation process where spins give up the energy absorbed through excitation to the surrounding molecular lattice of the tissue. It is called T1 recovery.
T2 decay is an irreversible loss of phase coherence due to spin-spin interactions on an atomic and molecular level.
Pulse sequences are mechanisms that permit refocusing of spins so that images can be acquired with different types of contrast.

8 T1 recovery

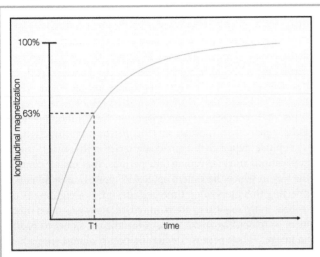

Figure 8.1 The T1 recovery curve.

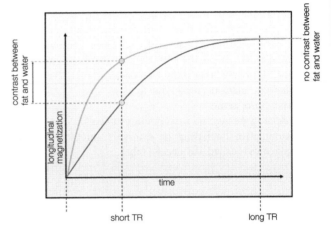

Figure 8.4 T1 recovery of fat and water.

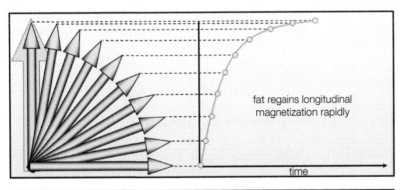

Figure 8.2 T1 recovery in fat.

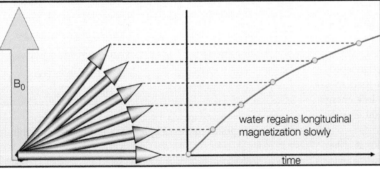

Figure 8.3 T1 recovery in water.

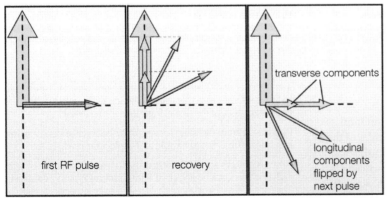

Figure 8.5 T1 contrast generation.

MRI at a Glance, Third Edition. Catherine Westbrook. © 2016 John Wiley & Sons, Ltd. Published 2016 by John Wiley & Sons, Ltd.
Companion website: www.ataglanceseries.com/mri

T1 recovery is caused by the exchange of energy from spins to their surrounding environment or lattice. It is called **spin lattice energy transfer**. As the spins dissipate their energy their magnetic moments relax or return to B_0; that is, they regain their longitudinal magnetization. The rate at which this occurs is an exponential process and it takes place at different rates in different tissues.

The **T1 recovery time** of a particular tissue is an intrinsic contrast parameter that is inherent to the tissue being imaged. It is a constant for a particular tissue and is defined as the time it takes for 63% of the longitudinal magnetization to recover in that tissue (Figure 8.1 and Table 8.1). The period of time during which this occurs is the time between one excitation pulse and the next or the **TR** (see Chapter 6). The TR therefore determines how much T1 recovery occurs in a particular tissue.

Table 8.1 Equations of T1 recovery.

Equations (if you like them)		
$Mz_t = Mz(1-e^{-t/T1})$	Mz_t is the amount of longitudinal magnetization at time t after the removal of the excitation pulse. Mz is full longitudinal magnetization. T1 is the T1 recovery time (ms) and is the time taken to increase the longitudinal magnetization by a factor of e.	This equation plots the size of the recovering NMV as a function of time after the removal of the excitation pulse and the T1 recovery time. When t=T1, 63% of the longitudinal magnetization recovers. When t=2xT1, 86% recovers and when t=3xT1, 95% recovers. It usually takes between 3 and 5 T1 recovery times for full recovery to occur.

T1 recovery in fat

T1 relaxation occurs as a result of spins exchanging the energy given to them by the RF pulse to their surrounding environment. The efficiency of this process determines the T1 recovery time of the tissue in which they are situated.

Due to the fact that fat is able to absorb energy quickly (see Chapter 5), the *T1 recovery time of fat is very short*; that is, spins dispose of their energy to the surrounding fat tissue and return to B_0 in a short time (Figure 8.2; Table 8.2).

Table 8.2 T1 relaxation times of brain tissue at 1 T.

Tissue	T1 relaxation time (ms)
Water	2500
Fat	200
CSF	2000
White matter	500

T1 recovery in water

Water is very inefficient at receiving energy from spins (see Chapter 5). *The T1 recovery time of water is therefore quite long*; that is, spins take a lot longer to dispose of their energy to the surrounding water tissue and return to B_0 (Figure 8.3; Table 8.2).

In addition, the efficiency of spin lattice energy transfer depends on how closely molecular motion of the molecules matches the Larmor frequency. If there is a good match between the rate of molecular tumbling and the precessional frequency of spins, energy is efficiently exchanged between hydrogen and the surrounding molecular lattice. The Larmor frequency is relatively slow and therefore fat is much better at this type of energy exchange than water, whose molecular motion is much faster than the Larmor frequency (see Chapter 5). This is another reason why fat has a shorter T1 recovery time than water.

T1 recovery is affected by the strength of the external magnetic field. The precessional frequency of spins within a tissue varies slightly, but efficient energy exchange due to molecular motion only occurs at the Larmor frequency. The Larmor frequency is proportional to B_0 and therefore T1 recovery takes longer as B_0 increases, because there are fewer molecules moving at relaxation-causing frequencies.

Control of T1 recovery

The TR controls how much of the NMV in fat or water recovers before the application of the next RF pulse.

A short TR does not permit full longitudinal recovery in most tissues, so that there are different longitudinal components in fat and water. These different longitudinal components are converted to different transverse components after the next excitation pulse has been applied. As the NMV does not recover completely to the positive longitudinal axis, they are pushed beyond the transverse plane by the succeeding 90° RF pulse. This is called **saturation**. When saturation occurs there is a contrast difference between fat and water due to differences in their T1 recovery times (Figures 8.4 and 8.5).

A long TR allows full recovery of the longitudinal components in most tissues. There is no difference in the magnitude of their longitudinal components. There is no contrast difference between fat and water due to differences in T1 recovery times when using a long TR. Any differences seen in contrast are due to differences in the number of protons or **proton density** of each tissue. The proton density of a particular tissue is an intrinsic contrast parameter and is therefore inherent to the tissue being imaged (see Chapter 6).

The key points of this chapter are summarized in Table 8.3.

Table 8.3 Key points.

Things to remember:
Fat has a short T1 recovery time.
Water has a long T1 recovery time.
T1 recovery is caused by spin lattice energy transfer. The efficiency of this process depends on the inherent energy of the tissue and how well the rate of molecular tumbling matches Larmor.
T1 recovery times are dependent on magnetic field strength. As field strength increases, tissues take longer to relax.
T1 contrast is controlled by the TR. For good T1 contrast, the TR must be short.

 Access the MCQs relating to this chapter on the book's companion website at www.ataglanceseries.com/mri

 Access Animation 2.1 relating to this chapter at www.westbrookmriinpractice.com/animations.asp

9 T2 decay

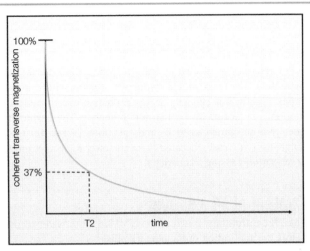

Figure 9.1 The T2 decay curve.

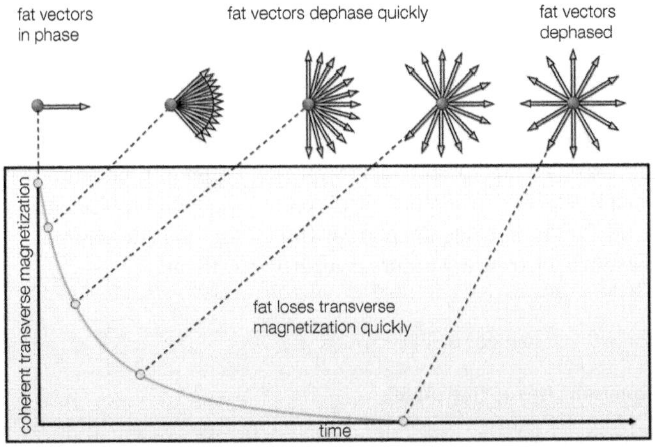

Figure 9.2 T2 decay in fat.

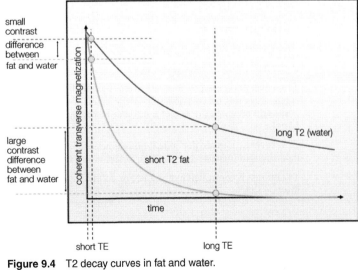

Figure 9.3 T2 decay in water.

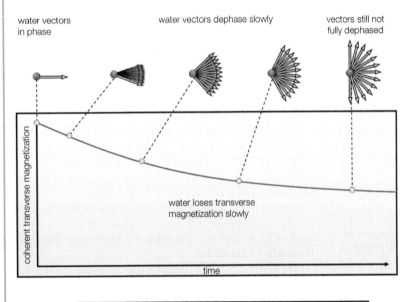

Figure 9.4 T2 decay curves in fat and water.

MRI at a Glance, Third Edition. Catherine Westbrook. © 2016 John Wiley & Sons, Ltd. Published 2016 by John Wiley & Sons, Ltd.
Companion website: www.ataglanceseries.com/mri

T2 decay is caused by the interaction between the magnetic fields of neighbouring spins. It is called **spin-spin**. It occurs as a result of the intrinsic magnetic fields of the nuclei interacting with each other. This produces a loss of phase coherence or dephasing, and results in decay of the NMV in the transverse plane. It is an exponential process and occurs at different rates in different tissues.

The **T2 decay time** of a particular tissue is an intrinsic contrast parameter and is inherent to the tissue being imaged. It is the time it takes for 63% of the transverse magnetization to be lost due to dephasing; that is, transverse magnetization is reduced by 63% of its original value (37% remains; Figure 9.1 and Table 9.1). The period of time during which this occurs is the time between the excitation pulse and the MR signal or the **TE** (see Chapter 6). The TE therefore determines how much T2 decay occurs in a particular tissue.

Table 9.1 T2 decay times of brain tissue at 1 T.

Equations (if you like them)		
$Mxy_t = Mxy\,e^{-t/T2}$	Mxy_t is the amount of transverse magnetization at time t (ms) after the removal of the excitation pulse. Mxy is full transverse magnetization. T2 is the T2 decay time (in ms) and is the time taken to reduce the transverse magnetization by a factor of e.	This equation plots the size of the decaying transverse magnetization as a function of time after the removal of the excitation pulse and the T2 decay time. When t=T2, 63% of the coherent transverse magnetization has decayed and 37% remains.

T2 decay in fat

T2 relaxation occurs as a result of the spins of adjacent nuclei interacting with each other. The efficiency of this process depends on how closely packed the molecules are to each other.

In fat the molecules are closely packed together so that spin-spin is efficient (see Chapter 6). *The T2 time of fat is therefore very short* (Figure 9.2).

T2 decay in water

In water the molecules are spaced apart so that spin-spin is not efficient (see Chapter 6). *The T2 time of water is therefore very long* (Figure 9.3).

Control of T2 decay

The **TE** controls how much transverse magnetization has been allowed to decay in fat and water when the signal is read.

A *short TE* does not permit full dephasing in either fat or water, so their coherent transverse components are similar. There is little contrast difference between fat and water due to differences in T2 decay times using a short TE.

A *long TE* allows dephasing of the transverse components in fat and water. There is a contrast difference between fat and water due to differences in T2 decay times when using a long TE (Figure 9.4).

T2 decay is affected by the strength of the external magnetic field. Spin-spin processes are more efficient when molecular motion occurs at the Larmor frequency. The Larmor frequency is proportional to B_0 and therefore T2 decay takes longer as B_0 increases, because there are fewer molecules moving at relaxation-causing frequencies.

It should be noted that fat and water represent the extremes in image contrast. Other tissues, such as muscle, grey matter and white matter, have contrast characteristics that fall between fat and water (Table 9.2).

Table 9.2 Equations of T2 decay.

Tissue	T2 decay time (ms)
Water	2500
Fat	100
CSF	300
White matter	100

Did you know?

The **stationary frame** of reference refers to the observer (i.e. you) viewing something moving. You and the room you are situated in are stationary and what you are observing moves.

The **rotating frame of reference** refers to the observer viewing this from a different perspective. Imagine you are the thing that moves, what would the room look like? You would appear stationary and the room would appear to move.

A good example of this is to imagine the NMV relaxing back to B_0. If you were to observe this from the stationary frame of reference, as the NMV relaxes it also precesses around B_0. If you are looking at this from the rotating frame, however, *you* become the NMV as if you 'ride along' with it. From this perspective the room moves around you (the NMV) and you just smoothly relax back to B_0. In other words, from the rotating frame of reference it is the room that precesses relative to the NMV, rather than the NMV precessing relative to the room (as with the stationary frame of reference).

The key points of this chapter are summarized in Table 9.3.

Table 9.3 Key points.

Things to remember:
Fat has a short T2 decay time.
Water has a long T2 decay time.
T2 decay is caused by spin-spin energy transfer. The efficiency of this process depends on how closely the molecules are packed together.
T2 decay times are dependent on magnetic field strength. As field strength increases, tissues take longer to dephase.
T2 contrast is controlled by the TE. For good T2 contrast, the TE must be long.

Access the MCQs relating to this chapter on the book's companion website at www.ataglanceseries.com/mri

Access Animation 2.1 relating to this chapter at www.westbrookmriinpractice.com/animations.asp

10 T1 weighting

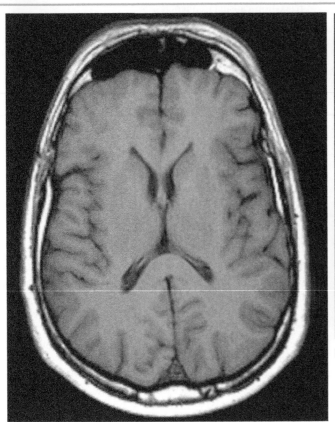

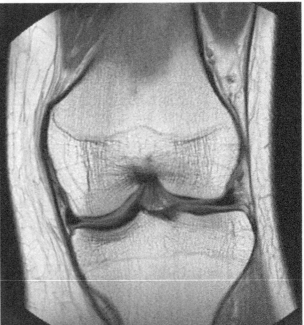

Figure 10.2 Coronal T1 weighted image of the knee.

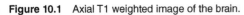

Figure 10.1 Axial T1 weighted image of the brain.

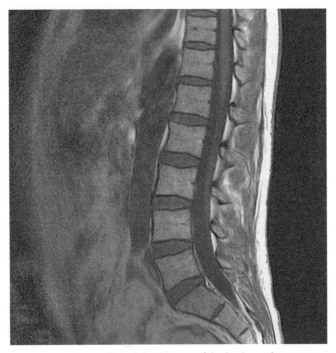

Figure 10.3 Sagittal T1 weighted image of the lumbar spine.

MRI at a Glance, Third Edition. Catherine Westbrook. © 2016 John Wiley & Sons, Ltd. Published 2016 by John Wiley & Sons, Ltd.
Companion website: www.ataglanceseries.com/mri

All intrinsic contrast mechanisms affect image contrast, regardless of the pulse sequence used. For example, tissues with a low proton density, and air, are always dark on an MR image, and tissues in which spins move may be dark or bright depending on their velocity and the pulse sequence used (see Chapter 46).

In order to produce images where the contrast is predictable, parameters are selected to weight the image towards one contrast mechanism and away from the others. This is achieved by understanding how extrinsic contrast parameters determine the degree to which intrinsic contrast parameters are allowed to affect image contrast. Extrinsic contrast parameters must be manipulated to accentuate one intrinsic contrast parameter and diminish the others. Flow and ADC effects are discussed later (see Chapters 26 and 46) and are not included in the following discussion. Proton density effects cannot be changed. T1 and T2 influences are manipulated by changing the TR and TE in the following way.

In a **T1 weighted image**, differences in the T1 relaxation times of tissues are accentuated and T2 effects are reduced. To achieve this, a TR is selected that is short enough to ensure that the NMV in neither fat nor water has had time to fully relax back to B_0 before the application of the next excitation pulse. The NMV in both fat and water is saturated. If the TR is long, the NMV in both fat and water recovers and the respective T1 relaxation times can no longer be distinguished (see Chapter 8).

A T1 weighted image is an image whose contrast is predominantly due to the differences in T1 recovery times of tissues. For T1 weighting, differences between the T1 times of tissues are exaggerated and to achieve this the *TR must be short*. At the same time, however, T2 effects must be minimized to avoid mixed weighting. To diminish T2 effects the *TE must also be short*.

In T1 weighted images, tissues containing a high proportion of fat, with short T1 relaxation times, are bright (high signal, hyper-intense), because they recover most of their longitudinal magnetization during the short TR period and therefore more magnetization is available to be flipped into the transverse plane by the next RF pulse and contribute to the signal (Table 10.1).

Tissues containing a high proportion of water, with long T1 relaxation times, are dark (low signal, hypo-intense), because they do not recover much of their longitudinal magnetization during the short TR period and therefore less magnetization is available to be flipped into the transverse plane by the next RF pulse and contribute to the signal (Table 10.1).

T1 weighted images best demonstrate anatomy, but also show pathology if used after contrast enhancement (Figures 10.1, 10.2 and 10.3).

Table 10.1 Signal intensities seen in T1 weighted images.

High signal	fat
	haemangioma
	intraosseous lipoma
	radiation change
	degeneration fatty deposition methaemoglobin
	cysts with proteinaceous fluid
	paramagnetic contrast agents
	slow-flowing blood
Low signal	cortical bone
	avascular necrosis
	infarction
	infection
	tumours
	sclerosis
	cysts
	calcification
No signal	air
	fast-flowing blood
	tendons
	cortical bone
	scar tissue
	calcification

Typical values

- TR: 400–700 ms (shorter in gradient echo sequences).
- TE: 10–30 ms (shorter in gradient echo sequences).

The principal pulse sequences that are capable of producing T1 weighted images are:

- spin echo (see Chapter 13);
- turbo spin echo (see Chapters 14 and 15);
- inversion recovery (see Chapter 16);
- incoherent gradient echo (see Chapter 21).

The key points of this chapter are summarized in Table 10.2.

Table 10.2 Key points.

Things to remember:

All intrinsic contrast parameters contribute to image contrast. Extrinsic contrast parameters are used to control how much influence each intrinsic parameter has on image contrast.

TR controls T1 contrast. TE controls T2 contrast.

To produce a T1 weighted image it is necessary to create contrast in which the differences in the T1 recovery times of the tissues dominate image contrast.

A short TR (e.g. 400 ms) combined with a short TE (e.g. 10 ms) maximizes T1 and minimizes T2 contrast respectively.

T1 weighted images are used for anatomy and pathology post contrast enhancement

Access the MCQs relating to this chapter on the book's companion website at www.ataglanceseries.com/mri

11 T2 weighting

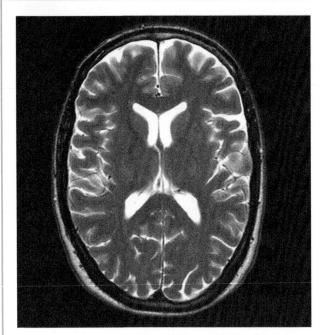

Figure 11.1 Axial T2 weighted image of the brain.

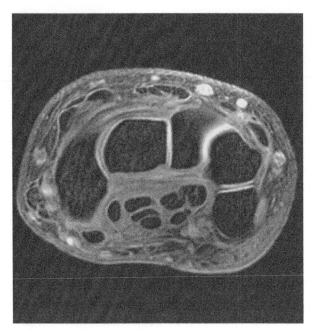

Figure 11.2 Axial T2 weighted image of the wrist.

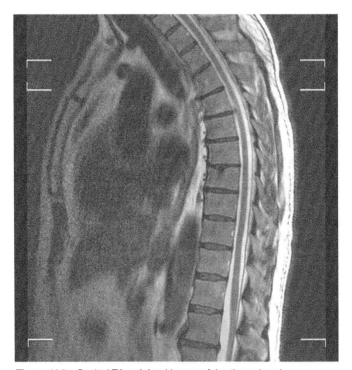

Figure 11.3 Sagittal T2 weighted image of the thoracic spine.

All intrinsic contrast parameters affect image contrast, regardless of the pulse sequence, TR and TE used. For example, tissues with a low proton density, and air, are always dark on an MR image, and tissues in which nuclei move may be dark or bright depending on their velocity and the pulse sequence used (see Chapter 46).

Therefore, parameters are selected to weight the image towards one contrast mechanism and away from the others. This is achieved by understanding how extrinsic contrast parameters determine the degree to which intrinsic contrast parameters are allowed to affect image contrast. Extrinsic contrast parameters must be manipulated to accentuate one intrinsic contrast parameter and diminish the others. Flow and ADC effects are discussed later (see Chapters 26 and 46) and are not included in the following discussion. Proton density effects cannot be changed. T1 and T2 influences are manipulated by changing the TR and TE in the following way.

In a **T2 weighted image** the differences in the T2 relaxation times of tissues are accentuated and T1 effects are reduced. To achieve this, a long TE is selected to ensure that the NMV in both fat and water has had time to decay. If the TE is too short, the NMV in neither fat nor water has had time to decay and the respective T2 times cannot be distinguished (see Chapter 9).

A T2 weighted image is an image whose contrast is predominantly due to the differences in the T2 decay times of tissues. For T2 weighting the differences between the T2 times of tissues are exaggerated, therefore the *TE must be long*. At the same time, however, T1 effects must be minimized to avoid mixed weighting. To diminish T1 effects *the TR must be long*.

Tissues containing a high proportion of fat, with a short T2 decay time, are dark (low signal, hypo-intense) because they lose most of their coherent transverse magnetization during the TE period (Table 11.1).

Tissues containing a high proportion of water, with a long T2 decay time, are bright (high signal, hyper-intense), because they retain most of their transverse coherence during the TE period (Table 11.1).

T2 weighted images best demonstrate pathology, as most pathology has increased water content and is therefore bright on T2 weighted images (Figures 11.1, 11.2 and 11.3).

Typical values

- TR: 2000+ ms (much shorter in gradient echo sequences)
- TE: 70+ ms (shorter in gradient echo sequences)

The principal pulse sequences that are capable of producing T2 weighted images are:

- spin echo (see Chapter 13)
- turbo spin echo (see Chapters 14 and 15)
- STIR/FLAIR (see Chapter 16)

The following pulse sequences produce T2* weighting that has similar characteristics in that water is bright. However, contrast in other tissues may be different.

- coherent gradient echo (see Chapter 20)
- balanced gradient echo (see Chapter 23)

The key points of this chapter are summarized in Table 11.2.

Table 11.1 Signal intensities seen in T2 weighted images.

High signal	water
	synovial fluid
	haemangioma
	infection
	inflammation
	oedema
	some tumours
	haemorrhage
	slow-flowing blood
	cysts
Low signal	cortical bone
	bone islands
	deoxyhaemoglobin
	haemosiderin
	calcification
	T2 paramagnetic agents
No signal	air
	fast-flowing blood
	tendons
	cortical bone
	scar tissue
	calcification

Table 11.2 Key points.

Things to remember:

All intrinsic contrast parameters contribute to image contrast. Extrinsic contrast parameters are used to control how much influence each intrinsic parameter has on image contrast.

TR controls T1 contrast. TE controls T2 contrast.

To produce a T2 weighted image it is necessary to create contrast in which the differences in the T2 decay times of the tissues dominate image contrast.

A long TR (e.g. 4000 ms) combined with a long TE (e.g. 100 ms) minimizes T1 and maximizes T2 contrast respectively.

T2 weighted images are used for pathology.

Access the MCQs relating to this chapter on the book's companion website at www.ataglanceseries.com/mri

12 PD weighting

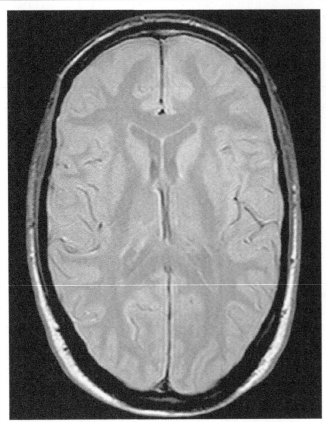

Figure 12.1 Axial proton density weighted image of the brain.

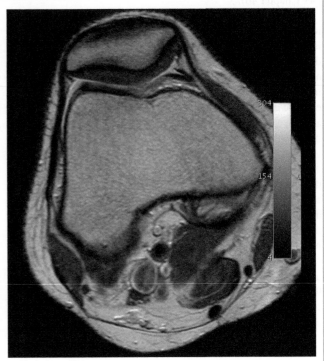

Figure 12.2 Axial proton density weighted image of the knee.

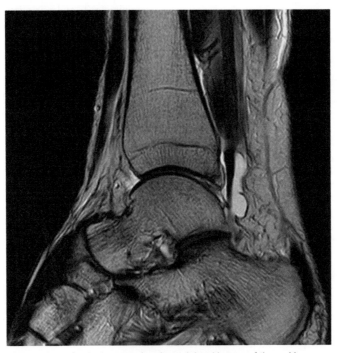

Figure 12.3 Sagittal proton density weighted image of the ankle.

MRI at a Glance, Third Edition. Catherine Westbrook. © 2016 John Wiley & Sons, Ltd. Published 2016 by John Wiley & Sons, Ltd.
Companion website: www.ataglanceseries.com/mri

All intrinsic contrast parameters affect image contrast, regardless of the pulse sequence, TR and TE used. For example, tissues with a low proton density, and air, are always dark on an MR image, and tissues in which nuclei move may be dark or bright depending on their velocity and the pulse sequence used (see Chapter 46).

Therefore, parameters are selected to weight the image towards one contrast mechanism and away from the others. This is achieved by understanding how extrinsic contrast parameters determine the degree to which intrinsic contrast parameters are allowed to affect image contrast. Extrinsic contrast parameters must be manipulated to accentuate one intrinsic contrast parameter and diminish the others. Flow and ADC effects are discussed later (see Chapters 26 and 46) and are not included in the following discussion.

In a **proton density (PD) weighted image**, differences in the proton densities (number of hydrogen protons in the tissue) are demonstrated. To achieve this, both T1 and T2 effects are diminished. Selecting a long TR reduces T1 effects and T2 effects are diminished by selecting *a short TE*.

A proton density weighted image is an image whose contrast is predominantly due to differences in the proton density of the tissues.

Tissues with a low proton density are dark (low signal, hypo-intense) because the low number of protons results in a small component of transverse magnetization (Table 12.1).

Tissues with a high proton density are bright (high signal, hyper-intense) because the high number of protons results in a large component of transverse magnetization (Table 12.1).

Cortical bone and air are always dark on MR images regardless of the weighting, as they have a low proton density and therefore return little signal. Proton density weighted images show anatomy and some pathology (Figures 12.1, 12.2 and 12.3).

Typical values

- TR: 2000 ms+
- TE: 10–30 ms

The main pulse sequences that are used to obtain PD weighting are:

- spin echo (see Chapter 13);
- turbo spin echo (see Chapters 14 and 15).

Other types of weighting

Flow and the ADC of a tissue also affect weighting, as they are intrinsic contrast mechanisms. Flow mechanisms can be used to weight the image specifically to flowing spins (see Chapter 48). Flow-related weighting is achieved in MR angiography techniques (see Chapters 47, 48 and 49). ADC-related weighting is achieved in diffusion weighting (see Chapter 25).

The key points of this chapter are summarized in Table 12.2.

Table 12.1 Signal intensities seen in PD weighted images.

High signal	CSF
	synovial fluid
	slow-flowing blood
	infection
	inflammation
	oedema
	cysts
	fat
Low or no signal	air
	fast-flowing blood
	tendons
	cortical bone
	scar tissue
	calcification

Table 12.2 Key points.

Things to remember:

All intrinsic contrast parameters contribute to image contrast. Extrinsic contrast parameters are used to control how much influence each intrinsic parameter has on image contrast.

TR controls T1 contrast. TE controls T2 contrast.

To produce a PD weighted image it is necessary to create contrast in which the differences in the proton densities of the tissues dominate image contrast.

A long TR (e.g. 4000 ms) combined with a short TE (e.g. 20 ms) minimizes T1 and T2 contrast respectively so that PD can dominate.

PD weighted images are used for anatomy and pathology.

13 Conventional spin echo

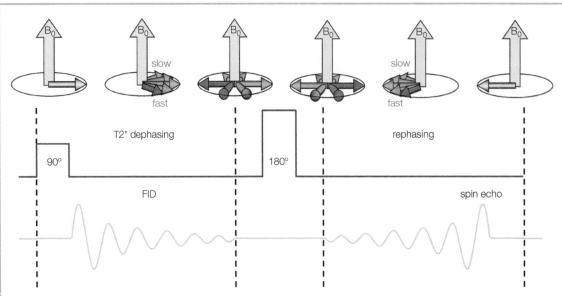

T2* dephasing

rephasing

90°

180°

slow

fast

slow

fast

FID

spin echo

Figure 13.1   180° RF rephasing.

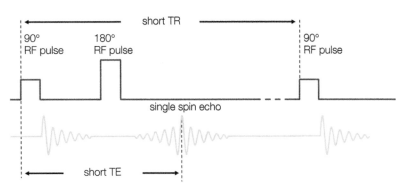

short TR

90°
RF pulse

180°
RF pulse

90°
RF pulse

single spin echo

short TE

Figure 13.2   Single-echo spin echo sequence.

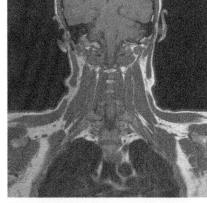

Figure 13.4   Coronal T1 weighted SE image of the brachial plexus.

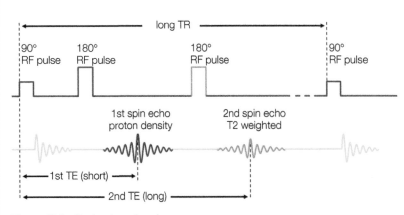

long TR

90°
RF pulse

180°
RF pulse

180°
RF pulse

90°
RF pulse

1st spin echo
proton density

2nd spin echo
T2 weighted

1st TE (short)

2nd TE (long)

Figure 13.3   Dual-echo spin echo sequence.

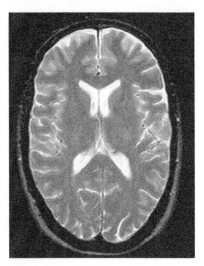

Figure 13.5   Axial T2 weighted SE image of the brain.

MRI at a Glance, Third Edition. Catherine Westbrook. © 2016 John Wiley & Sons, Ltd. Published 2016 by John Wiley & Sons, Ltd.
Companion website: www.ataglanceseries.com/mri

Pulse sequences are defined as a series of RF pulses, gradient applications and intervening time intervals. All pulse sequences contain these elements. They differ only in the way they are coordinated and timed.

Conventional spin echo (SE or CSE) pulse sequences are used to produce T1, T2 or proton density weighted images and are one of the most basic pulse sequences used in MRI. In a spin echo pulse sequence there is a 90° excitation pulse followed by a 180° rephasing pulse followed by an **echo**.

Mechanisms of CSE

After the application of the 90° RF pulse, the magnetic moments of the spins lose precessional coherence because of an increase or decrease in their precessional frequency caused by the magnetic field inhomogeneities. This results in a decay of coherent magnetization in the transverse plane and the ability to generate a signal is lost (see Chapter 7).

Magnetic moments that experience an increase in precessional frequency gain phase relative to those that experience a decrease in precessional frequency, which lag behind. Dephasing can be imagined as a 'fan' where magnetic moments that lag behind precess more slowly, and those that gain phase precess more quickly.

A 180° RF pulse flips magnetic moments of the dephased spins through 180°. The fast edge of the fan is now positioned behind the slow edge. The fast edge eventually catches up with the slow edge, therefore **rephasing** the spins (Figure 13.1).

The coherent signal in the receiver coil is regenerated and can be measured. This regenerated signal is called an **echo** and, because an RF pulse has been used to generate it, it is specifically called a **spin echo**.

Rephasing the spins eliminates the effect of the magnetic field inhomogeneities. Whenever a 180° RF rephasing pulse is applied, a spin echo results. Rephasing pulses may be applied either once or several times to produce either one or several spin echoes.

Contrast

CSE is usually used in one of two ways:
- A **single spin echo** pulse consists of a single 180° RF pulse applied after the excitation pulse to produce a single spin echo (Figure 13.2). This a typical sequence used to produce a T1 weighted set of images.

The **TR** is the length of time from one 90° RF pulse to the next 90° RF pulse in a particular slice. For T1 weighted imaging a short TR is used (see Chapter 10).

The **TE** is the length of time from the 90° RF pulse to the midpoint or peak of the signal generated after the 180° RF pulse; that is, the spin echo. For T1 weighted imaging a short TE is used (see Chapter 11).
- A **dual echo sequence** consists of two 180° pulses applied to produce two spin echoes. This is a sequence that provides two images per slice location: one that is proton density weighted and one that is T2 weighted (Figure 13.3). The first echo has a short TE and a long TR and results in a set of proton density weighted images (see Chapter 12). The second echo has a long TE and a long TR and results in a T2 weighted set of images (see Chapter 11). This echo has less amplitude than the first echo because more T2 decay has occurred by this point.

Typical values

Single echo (for T1 weighting)
- TR: 400–700 ms
- TE: 10–30 ms

Dual echo (for PD/T2 weighting)
- TR: 2000+ ms
- TE1: 20 ms
- TE2: 80 ms

Uses

Spin echo sequences are still considered the 'gold standard' (Table 13.1) in that the contrast they produce is understood and is predictable. They produce T1, T2 and PD weighted images of good quality and may be used in any part of the body, for any indication (Figures 13.4 and 13.5). However, due to relatively long scan times, PD and T2 weighted images are now usually acquired using fast or turbo spin echo (see Chapter 14).

Table 13.1 Advantages and disadvantage of conventional spin echo.

Advantages	Disadvantage
Good image quality Very versatile True T2 weighting Available on all systems Gold standard for image contrast and weighting	Long scan times

The key points of this chapter are summarized in Table 13.2.

Table 13.2 Key points.

Things to remember:
Spin echo sequences are characterized by 180°RF rephasing pulses that refocus the magnetic moments of spins to produce an echo.
T1, T2 and PD weighting are all achievable using conventional spin echo.
Conventional spin echois traditionally used to acquire one or two echoes to achieve T1, T2 or PD weighting.
Although quite old sequences, they are still considered the gold standard and can be used to image anatomy and pathology in all body areas.
Pulse sequence acronyms and acronyms for some imaging options are included in Appendix 3.

Access Animations 2.2 and 2.3 relating to this chapter at www.westbrookmriinpractice.com/animations.asp

14 Fast or turbo spin echo – how it works

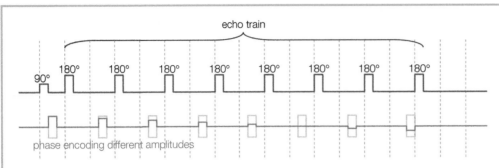

Figure 14.1 The echo train in TSE.

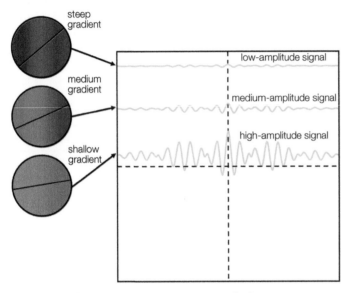

Figure 14.2 Phase encoding versus signal amplitude.

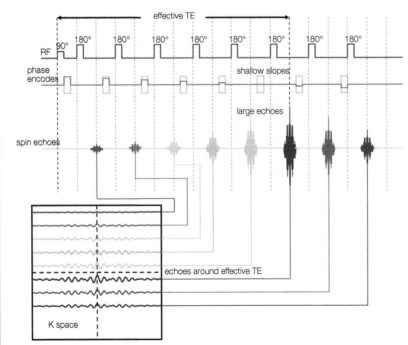

Figure 14.3 K space filling and phase reordering.

MRI at a Glance, Third Edition. Catherine Westbrook. © 2016 John Wiley & Sons, Ltd. Published 2016 by John Wiley & Sons, Ltd.
Companion website: www.ataglanceseries.com/mri

Fast or turbo spin echo (FSE or TSE) is a much faster version of conventional spin echo. It is sometimes called a rapid acquisition with relaxation enhancement (RARE) sequence. In spin echo sequences, one phase encoding only is performed during each TR (see Chapter 32). The scan time is a function of TR, NSA and phase matrix (see Chapter 36). One of the ways of speeding up a conventional sequence is to reduce the number of phase-encoding steps. However, this normally results in a loss of resolution (see Chapter 41). TSE overcomes this by still performing the same number of phase encodings, thereby maintaining the phase matrix, but more than one phase encoding is performed per TR, reducing the scan time.

Mechanism

TSE employs a train of 180° rephasing pulses, each one producing a spin echo. This train of spin echoes is called an **echo train**. The number of 180° RF pulses and resultant echoes is called the **echo train length (ETL)** or **turbo factor**. The spacing between each echo is called the **echo spacing**.

After each rephasing, a phase-encoding step is performed and data from the resultant echo is stored in a different line of K space (see Chapter 32 and Figure 14.1). Therefore several lines of K space are filled every TR instead of one line as in conventional spin echo. As K space is filled more rapidly, the scan time decreases.

Typically, 2 to 30 180° RF pulses are applied during every TR, although many more can be applied if required. As several phase encodings are also performed during each TR, several lines of K space are filled each TR and the scan time is reduced. For example, if a factor of 16 is used, 16 phase encodings are performed per TR and therefore 16 lines of K space are filled per TR instead of 1 as in conventional spin echo. Therefore the scan time is 1/16 of the original scan time (Table 14.1). The *higher* the turbo factor the *shorter* the scan time (Table 14.2).

Contrast

Each echo has a different TE and data from each echo is used to produce one image. This is different from CSE, where several echoes may be generated with a different TE but each echo is used to produce a *different* image. In TSE multiple echoes with a different TE are used to produce the *same* image. This would normally result in a mixture of weighting. In TSE this problem is overcome by using **phase reordering.**

In any sequence, each phase-encoding step applies a different slope of phase gradient to phase shift each slice by a different amount. This ensures that data is placed in a different line of K space.

The very *steep* gradient slopes significantly *reduce the amplitude* of the resultant echo/signal, because they reduce the rephasing effect of the 180° rephasing pulse. *Shallow* gradients, on the other hand, do not have this effect and the *amplitude of the resultant echo/signal is maximized* (see Chapter 33 and Figure 14.2).

When the TE is selected (known as the **effective TE** in TSE sequences) the resultant image must have a weighting corresponding to that TE; that is, if the TE is set at 102 ms a T2 weighted image is obtained (assuming the TR is long).

The system therefore orders the phase encodings so that those that produce the most signal (the shallowest ones) are used on echoes produced from 180° pulses nearest to the effective TE selected. The steepest gradients (which reduce the signal) are reserved for those echoes that are produced by 180° pulses furthest away from the effective TE. Therefore the resultant image is mostly made from data acquired at approximately the correct TE, although some other data is present (Figure 14.3).

On many modern scanners it is possible to reduce the magnitude of the RF rephasing pulse from 180° (e.g. 150°). Rephasing still occurs, because RF energy is delivered at the Larmor frequency, but, as the amplitude of the RF is less, SAR is reduced. Reduction in SAR allows for more slices for a given TR (see Chapter 54).

The key points of this chapter are summarized in Table 14.3.

Table 14.1 TSE time-saving illustrations.

Pulse sequence	Scan time
SE, 256 phase encodings, 1NSA	256 × 1 × TR = 256 × TR
TSE, 256 phase encodings, 1 NSA, ETL 16	256 × 1 × TR/16 = 16 × TR

Table 14.2 Equations of TSE scan time.

Equations (if you like them)		
ST = TR × Matrix(P) × NSA/ ETL	ST is the scan time (s) TR is the repetition time (ms) Matrix(P) is the phase matrix NSA is the number of signal averages ETL is the echo train length or turbo factor	This equation enables the scanner to calculate the scan time in TSE. The longer the echo train, the shorter the scan time, but may result in fewer slices per TR (see Chapter 15).

Table 14.3 Key points.

Things to remember:
Turbo or fast spin echo sequences involve applying the phase-encoding gradient multiple times in a TR period to varying amplitudes and polarity.
This means that multiple lines of K space are selected per TR. The number is equal to the echo train length (ETL) or turbo factor.
Multiple echoes are produced by multiple applications of an RF rephasing pulse and data from each echo is placed in a different line of K space.
Scan times are reduced by a factor equal to the turbo factor or ETL.
Image weighting is controlled by phase reordering so that data collected from echoes at or around the effective TE are placed in the signal and contrast areas of K space.
Pulse sequence acronyms and acronyms for some imaging options are included in Appendix 3.

Access the MCQs relating to this chapter on the book's companion website at www.ataglanceseries.com/mri

15 Fast or turbo spin echo – how it is used

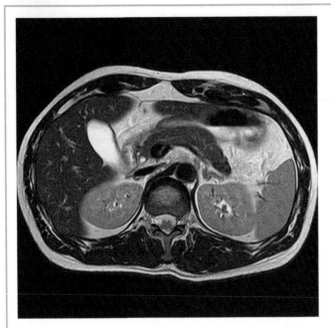

Figure 15.1 Axial T2 weighted TSE image of the abdomen.

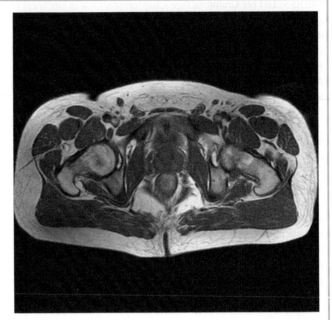

Figure 15.2 Axial T1 weighted TSE image of the male pelvis.

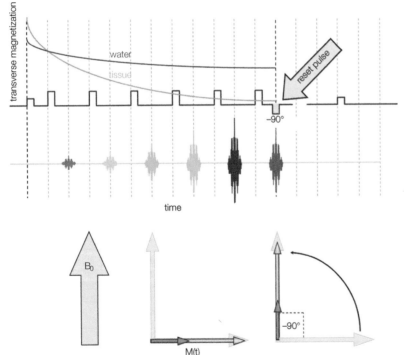

Figure 15.3 The fast recovery or 'DRIVE' sequence.

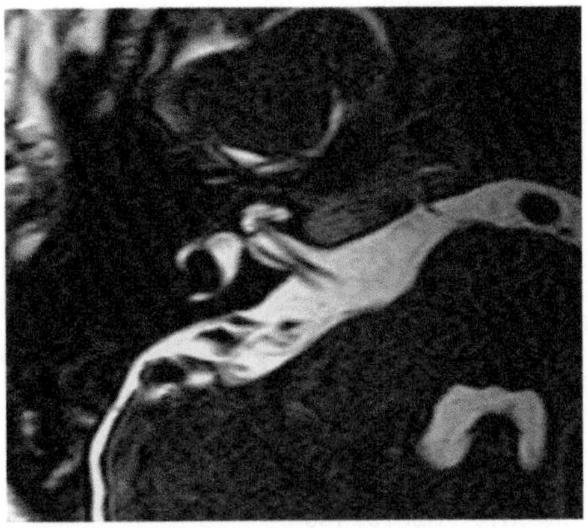

Figure 15.4 Fast recovery or 'DRIVE' image of the internal auditory meatus.

Due to different contrasts being present in the image, the contrast of TSE is unique. In T2 weighted scans, water *and* fat are hyper-intense (bright). This is because the succession of 180° RF pulses reduces the spin–spin interactions in fat, thereby increasing its T2 decay time (**J coupling**). Techniques such as STIR (see Chapter 16) and **chemical pre-saturation** (see Chapter 42) that suppress fat signal are therefore usually required to differentiate fat from pathology in T2 weighted TSE sequences.

Muscle is often darker than in conventional spin echo T2 weighted images. This is because the succession of RF pulses increases **magnetization transfer** effects that produce saturation (see Chapter 40). In T1 weighted imaging, CNR is sometimes reduced so that the images look rather 'flat'. It is therefore best used when inherent contrast is good.

When used with a very long echo train, TSE can sometimes result in images that are blurred. This is particularly the case when combined with a long echo spacing value. Echoes with a very long TE are likely to have low signal amplitude because of T2 decay. If data from these small echoes is mapped into the resolution lines of K space, image blurring can occur. This is usually only a problem with a very long echo train, however.

The number of slices is determined by the ETL and the echo spacing (see Table 15.1 and Scan Tip 1). Extending the TR lengthens the scan time, but this is more than compensated for by the use of long echo trains.

Table 15.1 Equations of TSE.

Equations (if you like them)		
$\text{N slices} = \dfrac{TR}{ETL \times E_S}$	N slices is the number of slices allowed per TR TR is the repetition time (ms) ETL is the echo train length or turbo factor E_S is the echo spacing (ms)	This equation shows how many slices are allowed in TSE and will be less than in conventional spin echo (see Scanning Tip 1).

Typical values

Dual echo
- TR: 2500–8000 ms (for slice number)
- Effective TE1: 17 ms
- Effective TE2: 102 ms
- Turbo factor 8: this may be split so that the PD image is acquired with the first four echoes and the T2 with the second four echoes

Single echo T2 weighting
- TR: 4000–8000 ms
- TE: 102 ms
- Turbo factor: 20+

Single echo T1 weighting
- TR: 600 ms
- TE: 10 ms
- Turbo factor: 4

Uses

TSE produces T1, T2 or proton density scans in a fraction of the time of CSE (Figures 15.1 and 15.2). Due to the fact that the scan times are reduced, phase matrix size can be increased to improve spatial resolution. TSE is normally used in the brain, spine, joints, extremities and pelvis. As TSE is incompatible with phase-reordered respiratory compensation techniques, it can only be used in the chest and abdomen with respiratory triggering, breath-hold or multiple NSA.

Systems that have sufficiently powerful gradients can use TSE in a single-shot mode (**SS-TSE**) or half Fourier single-shot TSE (**HASTE**). Both of these techniques permit image acquisition in a single breath-hold. In addition, using very long TEs and TRs permits very heavy T2 weighting (**watergrams**). An example of this technique is in gallbladder imaging, where only signal from bile in the biliary system is seen.

Table 15.2 lists some advantages and disadvantages of TSE.

Table 15.2 Advantages and disadvantages of TSE.

Advantages	Disadvantages
Short scan times	Some flow artefacts increased
High-resolution imaging	Incompatible with some
Increased T2 weighting	imaging options
Magnetic susceptibility	Some contrast interpretation
decreases*	problems
	Image blurring possible

* Also a disadvantage, e.g. haemorrhage not detected/delineated.

A modification of TSE that is sometimes called **fast recovery** or **DRIVE** adds an additional 'reset' pulse at the end of the TR period. This pulse 'drives' any residual magnetization in the transverse plane at the end of each TR back into the longitudinal plane (Figure 15.3). This is then available to be flipped into the transverse plane by the next excitation pulse. This sequence provides high signal intensity in water even when using a short TR and therefore a short scan time (Figure 15.4). This is because water has a long T2 decay time; therefore tissue with a high water content has residual transverse magnetization at the end of each TR. Hence this is the main tissue that is driven back up to the longitudinal plane by the reset pulse and is therefore the dominant tissue in terms of signal.

The key points of this chapter are summarized in Table 15.3.

Table 15.3 Key points.

Things to remember:
In turbo spin echo sequences fat remains bright in T2 weighted images due to J coupling. Fat suppression techniques are commonly employed.
The turbo factor or echo train length is an extrinsic contrast parameter unique to this sequence.
Short turbo factors or echo train lengths are necessary for T1 and PD weighting so that echoes with long TEs do not affect image contrast.
A long turbo factor or echo train length is needed for T2 weighting so that echoes with a long TE can affect contrast.
The longer the echo train, the shorter the scan time.
Turbo or fast spin echo has many applications in most body areas.

Access Scan Tip 1 and the MCQs relating to this chapter on the book's companion website at www.ataglanceseries.com/mri

16 Inversion recovery

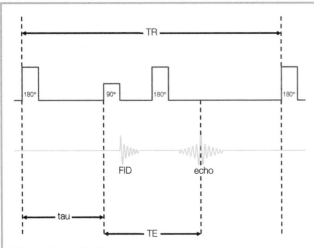

Figure 16.1 The inversion recovery sequence

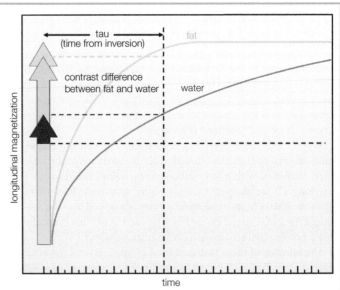

Figure 16.2 T1 weighting in inversion recovery

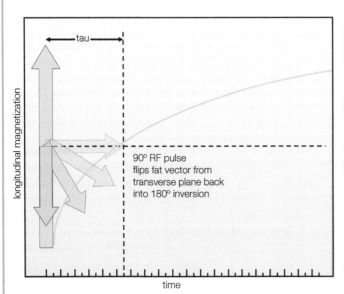

90° RF pulse
flips fat vector from
transverse plane back
into 180° inversion

Figure 16.3 How the use of short TI suppresses the signal from fat in a STIR sequence.

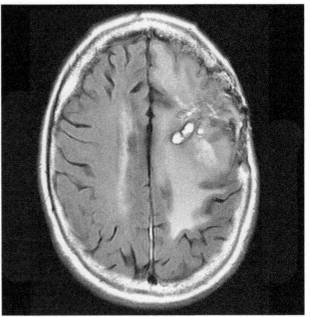

Figure 16.4 Axial T2 weighted FLAIR image of the brain

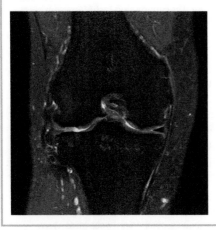

Figure 16.5 Coronal STIR of the knee.

MRI at a Glance, Third Edition. Catherine Westbrook. © 2016 John Wiley & Sons, Ltd. Published 2016 by John Wiley & Sons, Ltd.
Companion website: www.ataglanceseries.com/mri

Inversion **recovery** (IR) sequences were initially designed to produce very heavy T1 weighting. However, they are now mainly used in conjunction with a TSE sequence to produce T2 weighted images in which certain tissues are suppressed. Both are described here.

Mechanism

Inversion recovery is a spin echo sequence that begins with a 180° inverting pulse. This inverts the NMV through 180°. The TR is the time between successive 180° inverting pulses for a particular slice. When the pulse is removed, the NMV begins to relax back to B_0. A 90° pulse is then applied at time interval TI (time from inversion) after the 180° inverting pulse. A further 180° RF pulse is applied that rephases spins in the transverse plane and produces an echo at time TE after the excitation pulse (Figure 16.1).

Contrast

The **TI** is the main factor that controls weighting in IR sequences. If the TI is long enough to allow the NMV to pass through the transverse plane, the contrast depends on the degree of saturation that is produced by the 90° pulse (as in spin echo); that is, if the 90° pulse is applied shortly after the NMV has passed through the transverse plane, heavy saturation and T1 weighting result. A TI between 300 and 700 ms results in this type of heavy T1 weighting. Certain TI values result in the suppression of signal from tissues (Figure 16.2).

The TE controls the amount of T2 decay. For T1 weighting it must be short, for T2 weighting, long. The TR must always be long enough to allow full longitudinal recovery of magnetization before each inverting pulse. As a result, traditional inversion recovery sequences are associated with a very long TR and therefore long scan time.

Fast inversion recovery is a combination of inversion recovery and turbo spin echo. In this sequence the NMV is flipped through 180° into full saturation by a 180° inverting pulse. As in conventional inversion recovery, the TR is the time between each successive 180° pulse in a particular slice. At a time TI, the 90° excitation pulse is applied. However after this, multiple 180° rephasing pulses are applied to produce multiple echoes that are phase encoded with a different slope of gradient. As in turbo spin echo, multiple lines of K space are filled at each TR, thereby significantly reducing the scan time. This modification of inversion recovery is used in preference to the conventional sequence because, as the TR required for IR sequences must be increased in order to permit full recovery of the longitudinal magnetization, scan times are very long. Fast IR allows much shorter scan times to be implemented. The parameters used are similar to conventional IR, except that the ETL or turbo factor must be selected. This should be short for T1 weighting and long for T2 weighting.

With both sequence types a further modification of the TI allows suppression of signal from various tissue types.

STIR (short TI inversion recovery) uses a short TI such as 100–180 ms, depending on field strength. A TI of this magnitude places the 90° excitation pulse at the time that the NMV of fat is passing exactly through the transverse plane. At this point (called the **null point**) there is no longitudinal component in fat. Therefore the 90° excitation pulse produces no transverse component in fat and therefore no signal. In this way a fat-suppressed image results (Figure 16.3).

FLAIR (fluid attenuated inversion recovery) uses a long TI such as 1700–2200 ms, depending on field strength, to null the signal from CSF in exactly the same way as the STIR sequence.

Because CSF has a long T1 recovery time, the TI must be longer to correspond with its null point.

Typical values

T1 weighting
- TI: 300–700 ms
- TE: 10–20 ms
- TR: 2500+ ms
- Turbo factor: 4

STIR
- TI: 100–180 ms
- TE: 70+ ms (for T2 weighting)
- TR: 2500+ ms
- Turbo factor: 16+

FLAIR
- TI: 1500–2200 ms
- TE: 70+ ms (for T2 weighting)
- TR: 2500+ ms
- Turbo factor: 12–20

Uses

Inversion recovery is a very versatile sequence (Table 16.1) that is mainly used in the central nervous system (T1 weighting and FLAIR) and musculoskeletal system (STIR). The FLAIR sequence increases the conspicuity of peri-ventricular lesions such as MS plaques and lesions in the cervical and thoracic cord (Figure 16.4). STIR sequences are often called 'search and destroy' sequences when used in the musculoskeletal system, as they null the signal from normal marrow, thereby significantly increasing the conspicuity of bone lesions (Figure 16.5).

Table 16.1 Advantages and disadvantage of inversion recovery.

Advantages	Disadvantage
Versatile	Long scan times (conventional IR)
Good image quality	
Sensitive to pathology	

The key points of this chapter are summarized in Table 16.2.

Table 16.2 Key points.

Things to remember:
IR sequences are spin echo sequences with an initial 180° inversion pulse that saturates the longitudinal magnetization.
The TI determines the time between this and the 90° excitation pulse that follows. This parameter controls weighting in conventional and fast versions of this sequence.
When combined with an echo train as in TSE (see Chapter 14), scan times are reduced and this sequence is typically used to suppress the signal from either CSF (FLAIR) or fat (STIR).
A TI equivalent to the null point of either CSF or fat is used for this purpose. The ETL determines by how much the scan time is reduced.
Pulse sequence acronyms and acronyms for some imaging options are included in Appendix 3.

Access the MCQs relating to this chapter on the book's companion website at www.ataglanceseries.com/mri

Access Animation 5.1 relating to this chapter at www.westbrookmriinpractice.com/animations.asp

Gradient echo – how it works

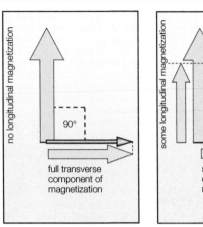

Figure 17.1 Flip angle vs signal amplitude.

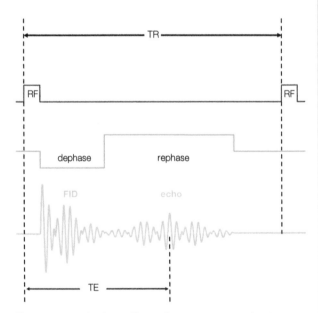

precessional frequency

speeds up   slows down

fast nuclei slow down
slow nuclei speed up

back in phase

Figure 17.3 How gradients rephase.

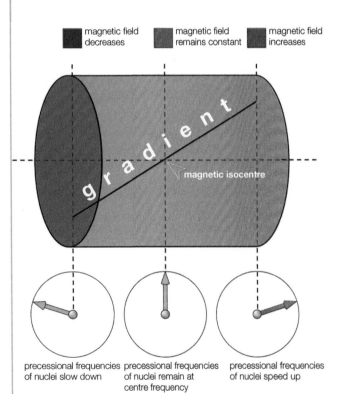

magnetic field decreases
magnetic field remains constant
magnetic field increases

magnetic isocentre

precessional frequencies of nuclei slow down

precessional frequencies of nuclei remain at centre frequency

precessional frequencies of nuclei speed up

Figure 17.2 How gradients alter field strength and frequency.

TR

RF   RF

dephase   rephase

FID   echo

TE

Figure 17.4 A basic gradient echo sequence showing how a bipolar application of the frequency-encoding gradient produces a gradient echo.

MRI at a Glance, Third Edition. Catherine Westbrook. © 2016 John Wiley & Sons, Ltd. Published 2016 by John Wiley & Sons, Ltd.
Companion website: www.ataglanceseries.com/mri

Gradient echo pulse sequences are sequences that use a gradient to rephase spins, as opposed to a 180° RF pulse used in spin echo sequences (see Chapter 13). They also use variable flip angles. Both of these strategies permit short scan times.

Mechanism

- The RF excitation and relaxation pattern used in gradient echo sequences consists of an RF excitation pulse followed by a relaxation period and the application of a gradient scheme to produce rephasing of spins.
- The magnitude and duration of the RF excitation pulse selected determine the **flip angle**; that is, the angle through which the NMV moves away from B_0 during resonance (see Chapter 5).
- Gradient echo sequences typically use flip angles that are less than 90° so that the longitudinal magnetization is not flipped as far as it is in spin echo sequences. As a result, full recovery in the longitudinal plane does not take as long as it does in spin echo sequences and therefore the TR can be shorter. This is one of the ways in which gradient echo sequences permit short scan times.
- A transverse component of magnetization is created, the magnitude of which is sometimes less than in spin echo, where all the longitudinal magnetization is converted to transverse magnetization. When a flip angle other than 90° is used, only part of the longitudinal magnetization is converted to transverse magnetization, which precesses in the transverse plane and induces a signal in the receiver coil. Therefore the signal to noise ratio (SNR) in gradient echo sequences is usually less than in spin echo sequences (see Chapter 39; Figure 17.1).
- The maximum achievable signal intensity and therefore transverse magnetization from a tissue using a particular TR are determined by the **Ernst angle**. However, in most gradient echo sequences the flip angle is chosen to maximize contrast between different tissues rather than generate maximum signal from every tissue (see Chapter 19).
- The magnetic moments within the transverse component of magnetization dephase, and are then rephased by a **gradient** scheme (Figures 17.2 and 17.3).
- A gradient causes a change in the magnetic field strength that changes the precessional frequency and phase of spins (see Chapter 53). This mechanism (called **rewinding**) rephases the magnetic moments so that the receiver coil receives signal. This signal is called a **gradient echo**, as a gradient rather than an RF pulse is used to create it (Figure 17.4).

In a gradient echo sequence, rephasing is performed by the **frequency encoding gradient** (see Chapter 30). The magnetic moments of the spins are dephased with a negative gradient pulse. The negative gradient slows down the magnetic moments of the slow spins even further, and speeds up the fast ones. This accelerates the dephasing process. The gradient polarity is then reversed to positive. The positive gradient speeds up the magnetic moments of the slow spins and slows down the fast ones. The magnetic moments of the spins rephase and produce a gradient echo (Figure 17.3). This bi-polar application of the frequency-encoding gradient is required so that the magnetic moments of spins are in phase at the same time that the system is reading frequencies in the gradient echo. This occurs in the middle of the application of the positive lobe of the frequency-encoding gradient or the **sampling window** (see Chapter 34).

Gradient rephasing is less efficient than RF rephasing. Gradient rephasing does not reverse the magnetic moments of spins that have been dephased from inhomogeneities in the main field. Gradient echo images therefore contain T2* effects such as increased noise and magnetic susceptibility artefact (see Chapter 45). Therefore T2 weighted gradient echo images are usually called T2* weighted images to reflect the presence of T2* effects such as field inhomogeneities. Gradient echo images are more sensitive to external magnetic field imperfections because T2* dephasing effects, produced by these inhomogeneities, are not eliminated by gradient rephasing (see Table 7.1).

Table 17.1 Key points.

Things to remember:

GRE sequences uses a gradient to rephase spins and usually flip angles less than 90°. Both of these strategies permit a shorter TE and TR than in spin echo.

Low flip angles mean that, as less longitudinal is converted to transverse during the excitation phase of the sequence, less time is required for relaxation. This is why a short TR can be used in GRE.

The speed of rephasing is increased using a gradient. A bipolar application of the frequency-encoding gradient enables spins to be rewound into phase in the middle of the sampling window when the system is reading the echo. The permits a short TE, which means that a shorter TR can be used for a given number of slices than in spin echo.

Although faster than RF rephasing, inhomogeneities are not compensated for in this type of sequence. Magnetic susceptibility artefacts therefore increase.

Pulse sequence acronyms and acronyms for some imaging options are included in Appendix 3.

Gradient rephasing is faster than RF rephasing and therefore these sequences use a shorter TE and TR than spin echo. As a result, scan times are short.

The key points of this chapter are summarized in Table 17.1.

 Access the MCQs relating to this chapter on the book's companion website at www.ataglanceseries.com/mri

18 Gradient echo – how it is used

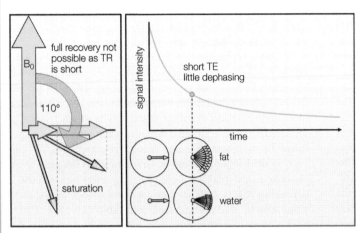

Figure 18.1   T1 weighting in gradient echo.

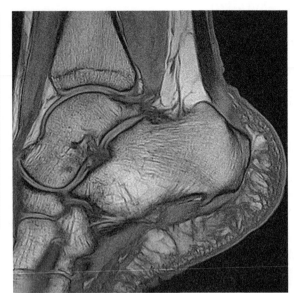

Figure 18.2   Sagittal T1 weighted gradient echo of the ankle.

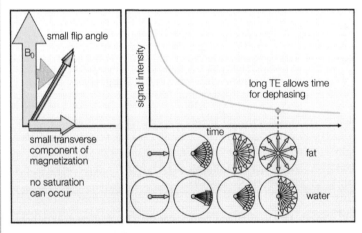

Figure 18.3   T2* weighting in gradient echo.

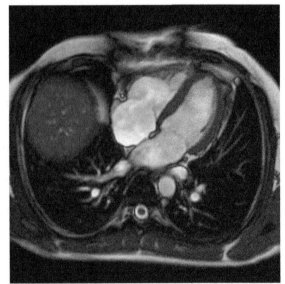

Figure 18.4   T2* weighted gradient echo of the four chambers of the heart.

MRI at a Glance, Third Edition. Catherine Westbrook. © 2016 John Wiley & Sons, Ltd. Published 2016 by John Wiley & Sons, Ltd.
Companion website: www.ataglanceseries.com/mri

Weighting in gradient echo sequences is controlled by several mechanisms. One of these relies on the manipulation of certain extrinsic contrast parameters (see Chapter 6). As in spin echo imaging, the TR controls T1 weighting. The TR used in gradient echo is usually much shorter than in spin echo. This normally increases saturation and therefore T1 weighting, especially if the flip angle is large. To overcome this, the flip angle is reduced to less than 90° so that the NMV is predominantly in the longitudinal plane. This prevents saturation so that the TR can be reduced.

In gradient echo sequences the TR and flip angle together control T1/proton density weighting. The TE determines the amount of T2 dephasing that occurs before the NMV is rephased and therefore the amount of T2 relaxation affecting image contrast. The longer the TE, the more T2* contrast in the image. As gradient rephasing is less efficient than RF rephasing at removing inhomogeneity effects, it contains more residual T2* effects than spin echo. As a result, the term T2* weighting is used in gradient echo imaging. In gradient echo sequences the TE controls T2* weighting.

Typical values

T1 weighting (Figures 18.1 and 18.2)
Use a TR and flip angle to produce maximum T1 effects. The flip angle must shift the majority of the NMV towards the transverse plane to produce saturation. *The flip angle must be large.*

The TR must not permit nuclei in the majority of tissues to recover to the longitudinal axis prior to the repetition of the next RF excitation pulse. Therefore *the TR must be short.*

Use a TE to produce minimum T2* effects. The TE should limit the amount of dephasing that occurs before the echo is regenerated. Therefore the *TE must be short.*

- TR: <50 ms (short)
- Flip angle: 60–120° (large)
- TE: <5 ms (short) (Table 18.1)

Table 18.1 Parameters used in gradient echo.

	TR	TE	Flip angle
T1 weighting	short	short	large
T2 weighting	long	long	small
PD weighting	long	short	small

T2* weighting (Figures 18.3 and 18.4)
The TE should permit maximum dephasing to occur before the signal is generated to produce maximum T2* effects. *The TE must be long.*

The flip angle must shift only a minimum of the NMV towards the transverse plane. Small flip angles ensure that the majority of the net magnetization components remain in the longitudinal axis to prevent saturation. *The flip angle must be small.*

The TR must be long enough to prevent saturation, but can be reduced without producing significant saturation because of the small flip angle.

- TR: >50 ms (long)
- Flip angle: <30° (small)
- TE: 15 ms (relatively long) (Table 18.1)

Proton density weighting
The TR and flip angle are selected to produce minimum T1 effects and a TE to produce minimum T2* effects. As a result, proton density predominates.

The *flip angle must be small* so that the majority of the NMV remains in the longitudinal axis and therefore saturation and T1 weighting are minimized.

The TR must be long to also minimize saturation and T1 effects.
The TE must be short to minimize T2* effects.

- TR: >50 ms (long)
- Flip angle: 5–20° (small)
- TE: 5 ms (short) (Table 18.1)

Uses
Gradient echo sequences have a variety of uses in clinical imaging. T2* weighted sequences are commonly used when a high signal intensity is required from water. Applications include white blood cardiac imaging (Figure 18.4) and spinal and joint imaging. T1 weighted sequences are often used in 3D techniques when it is necessary to view anatomy in multiple planes. In 3D imaging the scan time is multiplied by the number of slice locations and is therefore long compared to 2D acquisitions. It is therefore beneficial to use gradient echo sequences that are fast sequences in 3D imaging (see Scan Tip 6). Alternatively, the scan time saving of gradient echo sequences can be used to produce high-resolution T1 weighted images (Figure 18.2).

The key points of this chapter are summarized in Table 18.2.

Table 18.2 Key points.

Things to remember:

TR and flip angle control whether the NMV is saturated. Saturation is required for T1 weighting only.

TE controls T2* weighting.

For a T1 weighted gradient echo, the flip angle and TR combination must ensure that saturation occurs. The flip angle must be large and the TR short to achieve this. In addition, the TE must be short to minimize T2*.

For T2* weighted gradient echo, the flip angle and TR combination must prevent saturation. The flip angle must be small and the TR long to achieve this. In addition, the TE must be long to maximize T2*.

For PD weighted gradient echo, the flip angle and TR combination must prevent saturation. The flip angle must be small and the TR long to achieve this. In addition, the TE must be short to minimize T2*.

Access Scan Tip 6 and the MCQs relating to this chapter on the book's companion website at www.ataglanceseries.com/mri

19 The steady state

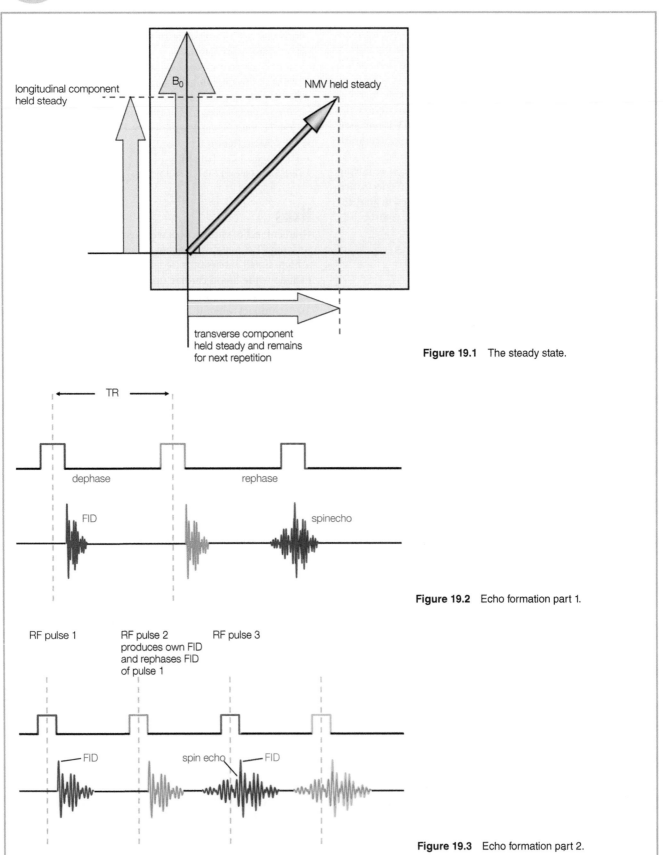

Figure 19.1 The steady state.

longitudinal component held steady

B_0

NMV held steady

transverse component held steady and remains for next repetition

TR

dephase

rephase

FID

spinecho

Figure 19.2 Echo formation part 1.

RF pulse 1

RF pulse 2 produces own FID and rephases FID of pulse 1

RF pulse 3

FID

spin echo

FID

Figure 19.3 Echo formation part 2.

The general definition of the **steady state** is a stable condition that does not change over time. For this to occur, any energy put into the system over time must equal any energy lost by the system in the same period.

In MR, energy is put into the patient via the RF excitation pulse applied to a slice every TR. The quantity of energy applied during excitation is determined by the amplitude and duration of the RF pulse and results in a flip angle of a certain magnitude (see Chapter 5). The amount of energy lost is determined by the TR period, as this is the time allowed for spin lattice energy transfer (see Chapter 7). To maintain the steady state, the TR and flip angle must be selected to ensure that the amount of energy given to the patient via excitation (as determined by the flip angle) more or less equals the amount of energy lost during relaxation (as determined by the TR).

The steady state is maintained when the TR is shorter than both the T1 and T2 relaxation times of all the tissues. If the TR were longer than this, unachievably large flip angles would be required to maintain the steady state. Most gradient echo sequences utilize the steady state, because the TR is so short that the fastest scan times are permitted. However, when a very short TR is selected, there is no time for the transverse magnetization to decay before the sequence is repeated again. The only process that has time to occur is T2*. Therefore the NMV does not really move between each TR and is held 'steady' (Figure 19.1). Because the transverse magnetization also does not have time to decay, its magnitude accumulates over successive TR periods. This **residual transverse magnetization** affects image contrast as the receiver coil detects its presence. Tissues containing a high proportion of water, with long T2 decay times, appear bright as they remain in the transverse plane longer than tissues with short T2 decay times. In addition to this, image contrast is determined by the T1 and T2 relaxation times of tissue. Tissues with similar relaxation times are brighter than those that are dissimilar. Hence water and fat are brighter than other tissues (Table 19.1).

Table 19.1 T1 and T2 relaxation times and signal intensity in the steady state at 1 T.

Tissue	T1 time (ms)	T2 time (ms)	T1/T2	Signal intensity
Water	2500	2500	1	↑
Fat	200	100	0.5	↑
Cerebral spinal fluid	2000	300	0.15	↓
White matter	500	200	0.2	↓

Echo generation in the steady state

As transverse magnetization does not have time to decay in the steady state, it builds up across successive TR periods and is rephased by each RF excitation pulse. Although the primary purpose of an excitation pulse is resonance, it will also rephase spins still present in the transverse plane and produce an echo if allowed to do so. This occurs because every RF pulse, regardless of its net magnitude, is able to rephase spins and produce an echo. Indeed, all RF pulses, regardless of their net magnitude (as determined by the flip angle), are able to excite and rephase spins. In spin echo sequences this secondary effect is destroyed, so that resonant (excitation) pulses only result in resonance, and rephasing pulses only result in rephasing the magnetic moments of spins to produce a spin echo. However, in the steady state these secondary effects are not eliminated, and hence every RF excitation pulse applied both results in resonance (and therefore an

FID when this pulse is removed) and also rephases any transverse magnetization to produce an echo. This occurs thus.

Every TR, an excitation pulse is applied. When the RF pulse is switched off, an FID is produced due to relaxation mechanisms (see Chapter 7). In the next TR period, another excitation pulse is applied, which also produces its own FID. However, it also rephases spins still in the transverse plane from the previous RF pulse and a spin echo results. Each RF pulse therefore not only produces its own FID, but also rephases the residual transverse magnetization produced from previous excitations. As the magnetic moments of spins take as long to rephase as they took to dephase, the echo from the first excitation pulse occurs at the same time as the third excitation pulse. This echo is called a **stimulated echo** (Figures 19.2 and 19.3).

This process continues throughout the sequence. In gradient echo sequences that utilize the steady state, there are therefore two signals available to produce the final gradient echo that is used to form the image:

• The **FID**, which is produced as a result of inhomogeneities. This contains mainly T1 weighted information, especially if the TE is short.
• The **stimulated echo**, which is the residual transverse magnetization, created across several TR periods, and contains mainly T2 weighted information, especially if the TE is long.

Most gradient echo sequences that use the steady state are described according to which of these signals they use to generate an image and therefore explain the contrast they produce.

The optimal flip angle in the steady state is determined by the relative signal intensity that a particular flip angle produces in tissues when using a very short TR. The **Ernst angle** is the flip angle that results in the highest signal intensity in a particular tissue for a particular TR (Table 19.2). Generally the shorter the TR, the lower the flip angle needed to produce maximum signal intensity in a tissue. However, to produce optimal contrast between tissues in the steady state, flip angles in the medium range are required. Therefore, to maintain the steady state the TR must be less than 50 ms and the flip angle between 30° and 45°.

Table 19.2 Ernst angle equation.

Equations (if you like them)		
Ernst = cos^{-1} [e (−TR/T1)]	Ernst is the Ernst angle in degrees TR is the repetition time (ms) T1 is the T1 relaxation time of a tissue (ms)	This equation determines the maximum signal intensity for a tissue with a certain T1 relaxation time at different TR values. When the flip angle is larger than the Ernst angle, saturation and therefore T1 contrast increase. When the flip angle is less than the Ernst angle, contrast relies more on PD.

The key points of this chapter are summarized in Table 19.3.

Table 19.3 Key points.

Things to remember:
The steady state is created when the TR is shorter than the T1 and T2 relaxation times of the tissues. Residual transverse magnetization therefore builds up over time.
The residual transverse magnetization is rephased by subsequent RF pulses to form stimulated echoes.
The resultant image contrast is therefore determined by the ratio of T1 and T2 in a particular tissue and whether the FID or the stimulated echo is sampled.

20 Coherent gradient echo

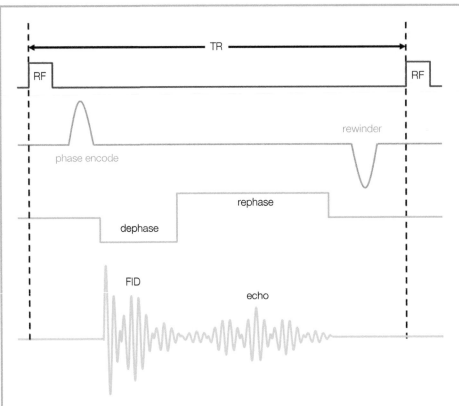

Figure 20.1 Coherent gradient echo sequence.

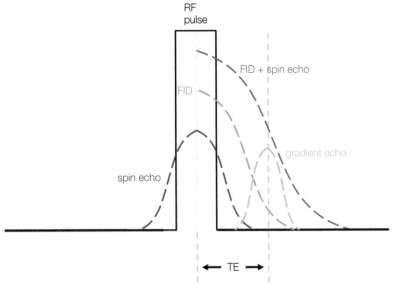

Figure 20.2 Echo generation in coherent gradient echo.

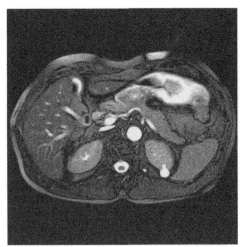

Figure 20.3 Axial coherent gradient echo image of the abdomen.

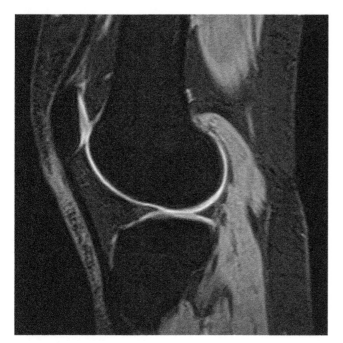

Figure 20.4 Sagittal coherent gradient echo image of the knee with tissue suppression.

The main types of gradient echo sequence are:
- **coherent** or rewind sequences (Table 20.1);
- incoherent or spoiled sequences;
- steady-state free precession;
- balanced gradient echo.

Table 20.1 Coherent gradient echo acronyms.

Philips	FFE
GE	GRASS
Siemens	FISP

Mechanism

This sequence is shown in Figure 20.1. It uses a gradient instead of a 180° RF rephasing pulse to rephase the magnetic moments of spins to form the echo. This means that a shorter TE is possible, because gradients rephase the magnetic moments of spins faster than RF pulses. However, inhomogeneities are not compensated for.

This sequence usually operates in the steady state by using a very short TR and a medium flip angle, so that there is residual transverse magnetization 'left over' when the next excitation pulse is delivered. The residual magnetization is rephased by each excitation pulse to produce a stimulated echo (see Chapter 19).

It employs a **rewinder** or **rephasing gradient** to amplify the effect of both the FID and the stimulated echo by maintaining their coherency. This gradient is a reversal of the phase-encoding gradient and means that coherency is preserved. This process is called **rewinding** and both the FID and the stimulated echo are used to produce the gradient echo that forms the resultant image (Figure 20.2).

Images contain both T1 and T2* contrast, but T2* effects dominate, especially if the TE is long. This is because the stimulated echo (that is formed from the residual transverse magnetization) is mainly made up of tissues containing a high proportion of water, with a long T2 decay time, because these tissues maintain their phase coherency longer than tissues with a short T2 decay time. These tissues (e.g. blood, CSF and synovial fluid) are therefore hyper-intense on the image. Coherent gradient echo sequences are thus often said to produce an angiographic, myelographic or arthrographic appearance.

Typical values

As coherent gradient echo sequences utilize the steady state, the TR and the flip angle must be at values to achieve this.

The TE determines how much T2* has occurred when the echo is regenerated. Coherent gradient echo sequences are primarily used to achieve T2* weighting using the following parameters:
- TR short (steady state): 35 ms
- Flip angle medium (steady state): 30°
- TE long (maximize T2*): 15 ms

Uses

The coherent gradient echo sequence is used when T2* weighted images (bright blood, synovial fluid or CSF) are required with good temporal resolution, for example:
- breath-hold T2* imaging (Figure 20.3);
- joint imaging (Figure 20.4);
- cine imaging of the heart;
- MR angiography (MRA);
- volume imaging with T2* weighting.

The advantages and disadvantages of this sequence are provided in Table 20.2. The sequence can also be used outside of the steady state (see Scan Tip 11).

Table 20.2 Advantages and disadvantages of coherent gradient echo.

Advantages	Disadvantages
Very fast scans	Reduced SNR in 2D acquisitions
Very sensitive to flow, so useful for angiography	Magnetic susceptibility increases
Can be acquired in a volume acquisition	Loud gradient noise

The key points of this chapter are summarized in Table 20.3.

Table 20.3 Key points.

Things to remember:
Coherent gradient echo is a steady-state sequence that utilizes a short TR and medium flip angle.
A reversal of the phase-encoding gradient rewinds all transverse magnetization so that its coherency is maintained.
Both the FID and the stimulated echo are sampled so that T1, T2* and PD weighting are possible.
This sequence is usually used with T2* weighting with a long TE to image water.
Pulse sequence acronyms and acronyms for some imaging options are included in Appendix 3.

 Access Scan Tip 11 relating to this chapter on the book's companion website at **www.ataglanceseries.com/mri**

21 Incoherent gradient echo

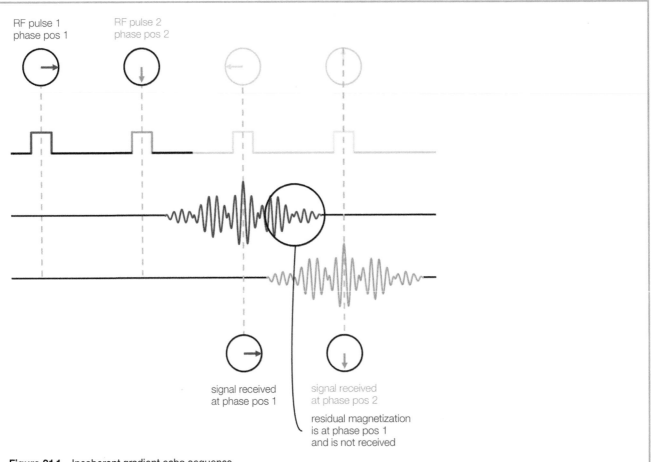

RF pulse 1
phase pos 1

RF pulse 2
phase pos 2

signal received
at phase pos 1

signal received
at phase pos 2

residual magnetization
is at phase pos 1
and is not received

Figure 21.1 Incoherent gradient echo sequence.

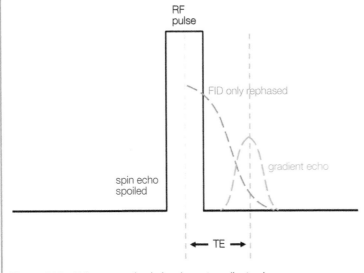

RF
pulse

FID only rephased

gradient echo

spin echo
spoiled

TE

Figure 21.2 Echo generation in incoherent gradient echo.

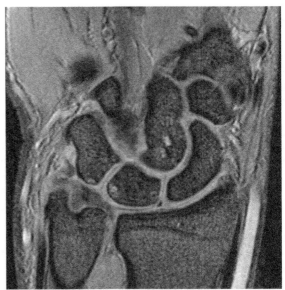

Figure 21.3 Coronal incoherent gradient echo from a 3D
data set.

MRI at a Glance, Third Edition. Catherine Westbrook. © 2016 John Wiley & Sons, Ltd. Published 2016 by John Wiley & Sons, Ltd.
Companion website: www.ataglanceseries.com/mri

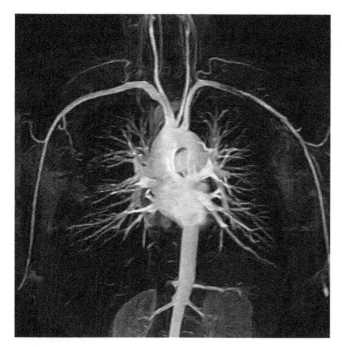

Figure 21.4 Coronal incoherent gradient echo acquired after gadolinium enhancement.

The main types of gradient echo sequence are:
- coherent or rewind sequences;
- **incoherent** or spoiled sequences (Table 21.1);
- steady-state free precession;
- balanced gradient echo.

Table 21.1 Incoherent gradient echo acronyms.

Philips	T1 FFE
GE	SPGR
Siemens	FLASH

Mechanism

This sequence is shown in Figure 21.1. It uses a gradient instead of a 180° RF rephasing pulse to rephase the magnetic moments of spins to form the echo. This means that a shorter TE is possible, because gradients rephase spins faster than RF pulses. However, inhomogeneities are not compensated for.

This sequence usually operates in the steady state by using a very short TR and a medium flip angle so that there is residual transverse magnetization 'left over' when the next excitation pulse is delivered. The residual magnetization is rephased by each excitation pulse to produce a stimulated echo (see Chapter 19).

The incoherent gradient echo sequence eliminates the stimulated echo, so that tissues with long T2 times are not allowed to dominate image contrast but T1/proton density contrast prevails. This is achieved by **RF spoiling**.

RF spoiling applies RF excitation pulses at different phases every TR, so that the residual transverse magnetization has different phase values than the transverse magnetization most recently created. The residual transverse magnetization is therefore differentiated from that most recently created because it has a different phase value.

The residual transverse magnetization and therefore the stimulated echo are not sampled. Only the FID is used to produce the gradient echo that forms the resultant image. Therefore images contain mainly T1 contrast (Figure 21.2).

Typical values

The incoherent gradient echo sequence utilizes the steady state, so the TR and the flip angle must be at values to achieve this.

The TE is as short as possible to minimize T2* effects. Incoherent gradient echo is primarily used for T1 weighting with the following parameters:
- TR short (steady state): 35 ms
- Flip angle medium (steady state): 35°
- TE short (minimize T2*): 5 ms

Uses

The incoherent gradient echo sequence should be used when T1 weighted images are required with good temporal resolution. For example:
- 3D volume acquisitions acquire data from a volume of tissue. A whole slab is excited (but not slice selected) and during the encoding process the slab is phase shifted into slices (**slice encoding**). As slice encoding is another form of phase encoding, the number of slices increases the scan time proportionally (see Chapter 36). 3D volume acquisitions are therefore quite lengthy scans and are often used with fast sequences (see Scan Tip 6). Volume acquisition allows very thin slices to be obtained at many slice locations. The data acquired can then be used to view the slab in any plane (Figure 21.3).
- 2D breath-hold T1 weighted sequences.
- Dynamic contrast enhanced images (Figure 21.4).

The advantages and disadvantages of this sequence are provided in Table 21.2.

Table 21.2 Advantages and disadvantages of incoherent gradient echo.

Advantages	Disadvantages
Fast scan times	Reduced SNR in 2D acquisitions
Can be used after gadolinium injection	Magnetic susceptibility increases
Can be acquired in a volume acquisition	Loud gradient noise
Good SNR and anatomical detail in 3D	

The key points of this chapter are summarized in Table 21.3.

Table 21.3 Key points.

Things to remember:
Incoherent gradient echo is a steady-state sequence that utilizes a short TR and medium flip angle.
RF spoiling ensures that residual transverse magnetization is not sampled.
Only the FID is sampled so that T1 weighting predominates.
Pulse sequence acronyms and acronyms for some imaging options are included in Appendix 3.

 Access Scan Tip 6 relating to this chapter on the book's companion website at **www.ataglanceseries .com/mri**

22 Steady-state free precession

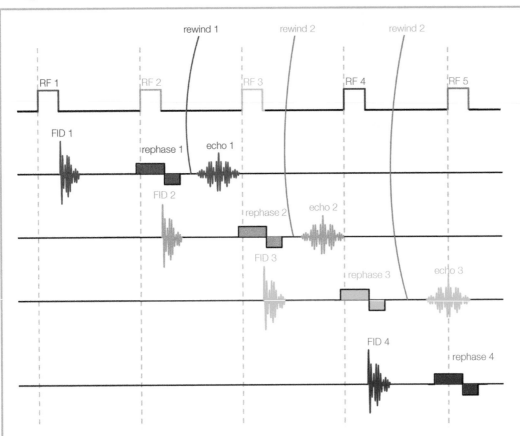

Figure 22.1 SSFP sequence.

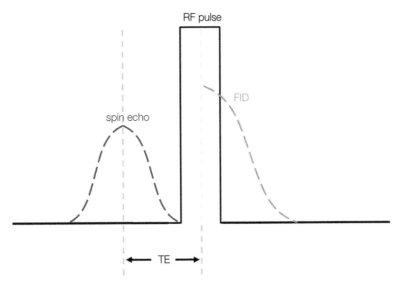

Figure 22.2 Echo generation in SSFP.

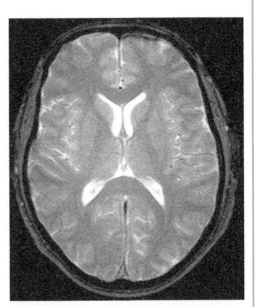

Figure 22.3 Axial SSFP image of the brain.

MRI at a Glance, Third Edition. Catherine Westbrook. © 2016 John Wiley & Sons, Ltd. Published 2016 by John Wiley & Sons, Ltd.
Companion website: www.ataglanceseries.com/mri

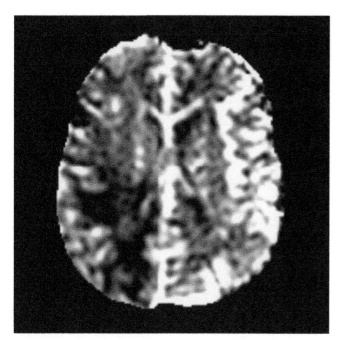

Figure 22.4 Perfusion imaging showing hyper-perfusion within oedema indicating recurrent tumour.

The main types of gradient echo sequence are:
- coherent or rewind sequences;
- incoherent or spoiled sequences;
- **steady-state free precession** or **SSFP** (Table 22.1);
- balanced gradient echo.

Table 22.1 Steady-state free precession acronyms.

Philips	T2 FFE
GE	SSFP
Siemens	PSIF

Gradient echo sequences do not demonstrate true T2 weighting, because the TE is never long enough to measure a tissue's T2 decay time. A TE of at least 70 ms is required to demonstrate true T2 weighting, and in gradient echo sequences the TE is rarely higher than 15 ms. SSFP is a steady-state sequence that obtains images that have a sufficiently long TE to measure T2 decay when using the steady state while still using a short TR. This is achieved in the following manner.

Mechanism

This sequence is shown in Figure 22.1. It uses a gradient instead of a 180° RF rephasing pulse to rephase the echo. It usually operates in the steady state by using a very short TR and a medium flip angle, so that there is residual transverse magnetization 'left over' when the next excitation pulse is delivered. Each RF pulse not only excites spins in a slice, it also rephases the residual transverse magnetization still present from the previous excitation and produces a stimulated echo (see Chapter 19).

As the magnetic moments of spins take as long to rephase after a 180° RF rephasing pulse as they took to dephase before it, the stimulated echo occurs at the same time as the third excitation pulse. In SSFP this stimulated echo is sampled. However, in order to do this it must be repositioned away from the excitation pulse, as RF cannot be transmitted and received at the same time.

To achieve this, a **rewinder** gradient is used to speed up the rephasing process after the RF rephasing has begun. Rewinding

repositions the echo so that it occurs sooner than usual and it no longer occurs at the same time as an excitation pulse. In this way, the stimulated echo is received and data from it is collected. This data is used to form the image (Figure 22.2). The resultant echo demonstrates more true T2 weighting than conventional gradient echo sequences. This is because the TE is now longer than the TR. In SSFP, there are usually two time periods to consider:
- the **actual TE** (time between the stimulated echo and the next excitation pulse);
- the **effective TE** (time from the stimulated echo to the excitation pulse that created it. This is the TE that determines the T2 weighting of the image). Therefore:

the effective TE = (2 × TR) minus actual TE

This means that the effective TE is longer than the TR and is long enough to measure the true T2. From the equation above it can be seen that the shorter the actual TE, the higher the effective TE and hence increased T2 weighting.

Typical values

- Flip angle: 30–45°
- TR: <50 ms
- TE (actual): 7 ms

Uses

SSFP sequences are used to rapidly acquire images that demonstrate true T2 weighting (Figure 22.3). With the advent of turbo spin echo, however, this sequence is not usually used for this purpose. But the principle of echo shifting (moving an echo to increase the effective TE) in conjunction with a short TR is used in many techniques, including perfusion imaging (see Figure 22.4 and Chapter 25).

The advantages and disadvantages of this sequence are provided in Table 22.2.

Table 22.2 Advantages and disadvantages of SSFP.

Advantages	Disadvantages
Fast scan times	Reduced SNR in 2D acquisitions
Truer T2 than in conventional gradient echo	Loud gradient noise
Can be acquired in a volume acquisition	Susceptible to artefacts
Good SNR and anatomical detail in 3D	Image quality can be poor

The key points of this chapter are summarized in Table 22.3.

Table 22.3 Key points.

Things to remember:

Incoherent gradient echo is a steady-state sequence that utilizes a short TR and medium flip angle.

Rephasing of the stimulated echo is initiated with an RF pulse, but the echo is repositioned by a rewinder gradient.

Only the stimulated echo is sampled and due to its repositioning the TE of this echo is long enough to include T2 rather than T2* contrast.

Pulse sequence acronyms and acronyms for some imaging options are included in Appendix 3.

23 Balanced gradient echo

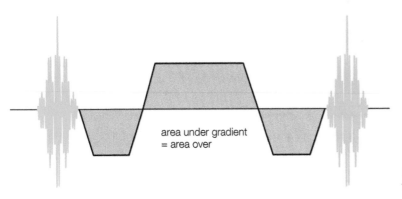

area under gradient
= area over

Figure 23.1 Balanced gradient echo scheme in the balanced gradient echo sequence.

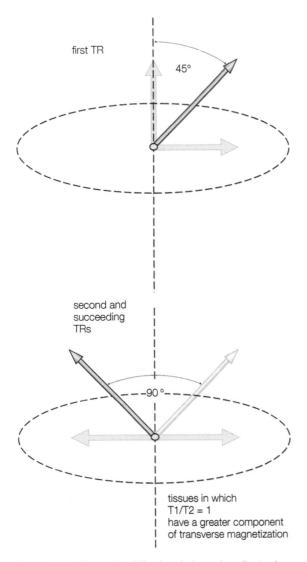

first TR

45°

second and
succeeding
TRs

90°

tissues in which
T1/T2 = 1
have a greater component
of transverse magnetization

Figure 23.2 Alternating RF pulses balanced gradient echo.

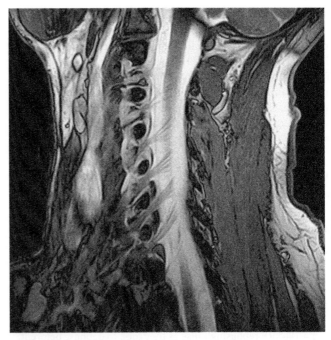

Figure 23.3 Sagittal oblique balanced gradient echo of the cervical cord showing nerve roots and peripheral nerves.

MRI at a Glance, Third Edition. Catherine Westbrook. © 2016 John Wiley & Sons, Ltd. Published 2016 by John Wiley & Sons, Ltd.
Companion website: www.ataglanceseries.com/mri

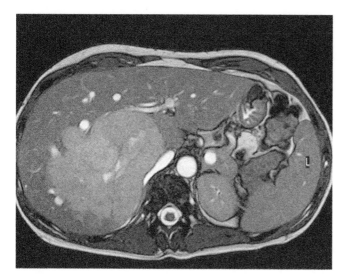

Figure 23.4 Axial balanced gradient echo of the abdomen.

The main types of gradient echo sequence are:
- coherent or rewind sequences;
- incoherent or spoiled sequences;
- steady-state free precession;
- **balanced gradient echo** (Table 23.1).

Table 23.1 Balanced gradient echo acronyms.

Philips	BFFE
GE	FIESTA
Siemens	True FISP

This sequence was developed to:
- reduce flow artefacts from high signal intensity areas;
- increase SNR and CNR in gradient echo sequences.

To reduce flow artefacts it is important to reduce the TR to a minimum, so that there is less time for spins to exit the slice (see Chapter 46). The SNR is increased by increasing the flip angle (see Chapter 39). However, combining a very short TR with a large flip angle results in saturation and therefore an increase in T1 weighting. The purpose of balanced gradient echo is to use a large flip angle (that increases SNR) with a very short TR (that reduces flow artefacts) while at the same time reducing saturation and increasing T2* weighting. This is achieved in the following manner.

Mechanism

A flow-compensated balanced gradient system is used on all three gradients to maintain coherency in flowing spins, thereby increasing their signal intensity (see Figure 23.1 and Chapter 43).

A large flip angle (e.g. 90°) is selected, but in the first TR only half this flip angle is applied (e.g. 45°). The RF excitation pulse creates transverse magnetization at a particular phase position in the transverse plane.

In the second TR period a second excitation pulse is applied that creates transverse magnetization 180° out of phase with the transverse magnetization created in the first TR period. This is achieved by applying the second RF pulse at a flip angle of −90° to the first excitation pulse (Figure 23.2).

Saturation does not occur, because the transverse magnetization created in the second TR period does not add to that created in the first TR period, since it has a different phase position on the transverse plane.

This pattern is repeated throughout the sequence. Every TR the phase of the transverse magnetization is changed by alternating the flip angle between +90° and −90°, therefore creating transverse magnetization at a different phase each time. Saturation is thereby prevented despite using a large flip angle and a very short TR, and T2* weighting can predominate. Large flip angles maximize SNR. A very short TR is used to minimize flow artefacts, as there is less time for spins to exit the slice.

Typical values

- Flip angle: 90°
- TE: 15 ms
- TR: <10 ms

Uses

Although this sequence was primarily developed for use in cardiac imaging, it is also important whenever T2* weighted images are required in areas where flow causes motion artefact. Commonly this sequence is used in the central nervous system to reduce flow from CSF, for instance the internal auditory meatus (IAM) and the cervical spine (Figure 23.3). However, it is also used in the abdominal system to reduce flow artefacts in the biliary and circulatory systems (Figure 23.4). As the TR is so short, this sequence provides excellent temporal resolution and is also useful in volume imaging.

The advantages and disadvantages of this sequence are provided in Table 23.2.

Table 23.2 Advantages and disadvantages of balanced gradient echo.

Advantages	Disadvantages
Fast scan times	Reduced SNR in 2D acquisitions
Reduced artefact from flow	Loud gradient noise
Good SNR and anatomical detail in 3D	Susceptible to artefacts
Images demonstrate good contrast	Requires high-performance gradients

The key points of this chapter are summarized in Table 23.3.

Table 23.3 Key points.

Things to remember:
Balanced gradient echo is a steady-state sequence in which longitudinal magnetization is maintained during the acquisition, thereby preventing saturation.
This is achieved by altering the phase angle of each RF excitation pulse every TR.
A balanced gradient scheme is used on all three gradients to correct for flow artefacts.
Pulse sequence acronyms and acronyms for some imaging options are included in Appendix 3.

24 Ultrafast sequences

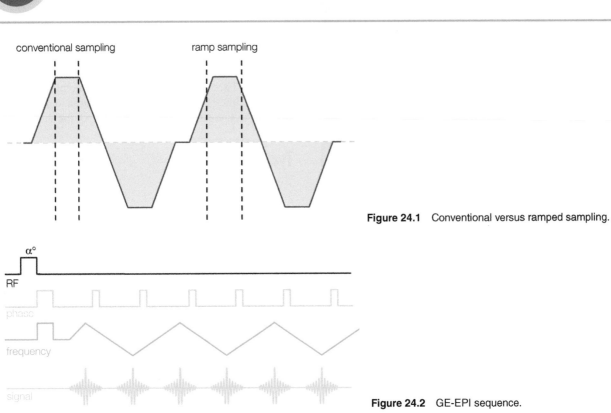

conventional sampling   ramp sampling

Figure 24.1 Conventional versus ramped sampling.

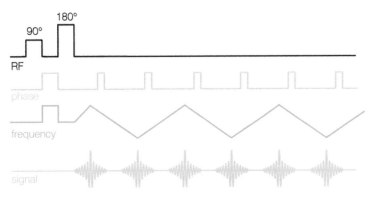

α°

RF

phase

frequency

signal

Figure 24.2 GE-EPI sequence.

180°

90°

RF

phase

frequency

signal

Figure 24.3 SE-EPI sequence.

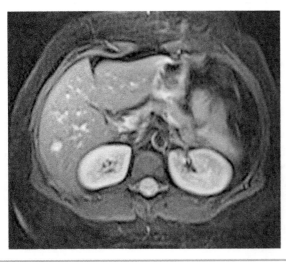

Figure 24.4 Axial SE-EPI of the abdomen.

Turbo gradient echo

Very fast pulse sequences include faster versions of coherent and incoherent gradient echo sequences or combinations of both (**hybrids**). Faster scan times are achieved in the following ways:
- applying only a portion of the RF excitation pulse, so that it takes much less time to apply and switch off;
- reading only a proportion of the echo (**partial echo**);
- using asymmetric gradients, which are faster to apply than conventional balanced gradients;
- sampling frequencies while the frequency-encoding gradient is still rising (**ramped sampling**) (see Figure 24.1 and Scan Tip 5);
- filling K space in a single shot or in segments (see Chapter 38).

These measures ensure that the TE and TR are very short. A TE as low as 1 ms and a TR as low as 5 ms can be achieved in this manner, enabling a 3D slab to be imaged in a single breath-hold. In addition, many ultrafast sequences use extra pulses applied before the pulse sequence begins to premagnetize the tissue. In this way a certain contrast can be obtained. Premagnetization is usually achieved by applying a 180° RF pulse before the pulse sequence begins. This inverts the NMV into full saturation and, at a specified delay time, the pulse sequence itself begins. This can be used to null signal from certain organs and tissues and is similar to inversion recovery. It is sometimes known as a **magnetization prepared** sequence.

Weighting is achieved by applying all the shallowest phase-encoding gradients first, and leaving the steep ones until the end of the pulse sequence. In this way, the effect of the premagnetization prevails as, when it is dominant, the central phase encodings (that produce the greatest signal amplitudes and determine the weighting of the sequence) are performed (see Chapter 38). By the end of the sequence, the premagnetization has decayed and this is when the low-signal amplitudes are acquired.

Echo planar imaging

Echo planar imaging or **EPI** is an MR acquisition method that either fills all the lines of K space in a single repetition (single shot – SS) or in multiple sections (multishot – MS). In order to achieve this, multiple echoes are generated and each is phase encoded by a different slope of gradient to fill all the required lines of K space. Echoes are generated by oscillation of the frequency-encoding gradient and therefore K space is filled with data acquired from multiple gradient echoes. In order to fill all of K space in this way, the readout and phase-encoding gradients must rapidly switch on and off (see Chapter 37). This technique is called **SS-EPI** or **MS-EPI**, depending on whether K space is filled in one repetition or several. There are many types of EPI sequence (Table 24.1):
- **GE-EPI** uses a variable flip angle followed by EPI readout in K space (Figure 24.2).
- **SE-EPI** uses 90°/180° followed by EPI readout in K space (Figures 24.3 and 24.4).
- **IR-EPI** uses 180°/90°/180° followed by EPI readout in K space.

Table 24.1 Single and multishot methods.

Sequence	Mechanism	Readout	Time
SS or MS-FSE	90/180 echo train	spin echo	min/s
SS or MS SE-EPI	90/180	gradient echo	s/subs
SS or MS GE-EPI	variable flip	gradient echo	s/subs
SS or MS IR-EPI	189/90/180	gradient echo	s/subs

Note: Single shot or multishot techniques in which spin echoes are generated by 180° rephasing pulses instead of gradient echoes are called **single shot or multishot turbo spin echo** (**SS-TSE** or **MS-TSE**; see Chapter 14).

Gradient rephasing as used by SS-EPI or MS-EPI techniques is much faster than RF rephasing (as used by SS-TSE or MS-TSE) and involves no RF deposition to the patient, but requires high-speed gradients. However, artefacts are more abundant, as inhomogeneity effects are not compensated for by gradient rephasing. EPI sequences place exceptional strains on the gradients and therefore gradient modifications are required (Table 24.2).

Table 24.2 Advantages and disadvantages of EPI.

Advantages	Disadvantages
Very fast scan times	Chemical shift artefact is common
Reduced artefact from respiratory and cardiac motion	Peripheral nerve stimulation due to fast switching of gradients
All three types of weighting can be achieved	Susceptible to artefacts
Functional information acquired	
Scan time savings can be used to improve phase resolution	

Typical values

Either proton density or T2 weighting is achieved by selecting either a short or long effective TE, which corresponds to the time interval between the excitation pulse and when the centre of K space is filled. In single shot techniques, as there is only one excitation pulse, there is no repetition and as a result the TR is said to equal infinity; that is, it is infinitely long. T1 weighting is only possible by applying an inverting pulse prior to the excitation pulse to produce saturation.

Uses

- Diffusion weighted imaging (see Chapter 25).
- Perfusion imaging (see Chapter 25).
- Functional imaging (see Chapter 26).
- Real-time cardiac imaging.
- Interventional techniques.
- Breath-hold techniques.

The advantages and disadvantages of this sequence are provided in Table 24.2.

The key points of this chapter are summarized in Table 24.3.

Table 24.3 Key points.

Things to remember:

Fast or turbo versions of the traditional gradient echo sequences use strategies such as ramped sampling and fractional echo to reduce scan times.

EPI is a method of filling K space in a single or multiple shot by oscillating the frequency-encoding gradient and reading the resultant gradient echoes.

Ultrafast sequences are commonly used to acquire functional rather than anatomical information.

Pulse sequence acronyms and acronyms for some imaging options are included in Appendix 3.

 Access Scan Tip 5 relating to this chapter on the book's companion website at **www.ataglanceseries.com/mri**

25 Diffusion and perfusion imaging

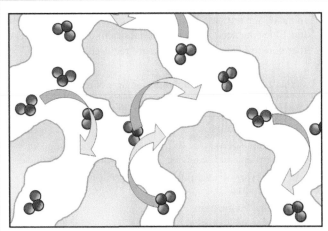

freely diffusing water

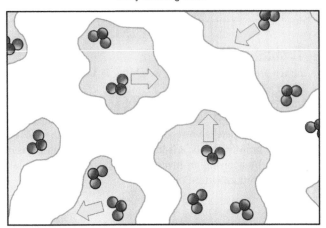

restricted water

Figure 25.1   Free and restricted diffusion.

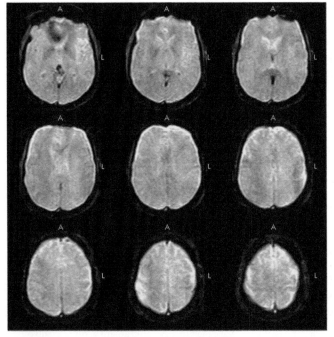

Figure 25.3   DTI of the brain showing white matter tracts.

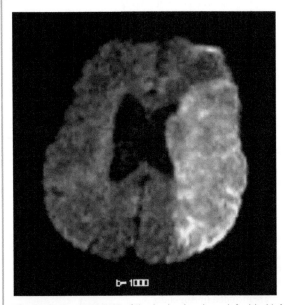

b= 1000

Figure 25.2   Axial DWI of the brain showing a left-sided infarct.

Figure 25.4   Set of perfusion images of the brain.

MRI at a Glance, Third Edition. Catherine Westbrook. © 2016 John Wiley & Sons, Ltd. Published 2016 by John Wiley & Sons, Ltd.
Companion website: www.ataglanceseries.com/mri

Diffusion weighted imaging

Diffusion is a term used to describe moving molecules due to random thermal motion. It is also called **Brownian motion.** This motion is restricted by boundaries such as ligaments, membranes and macromolecules and by pathology. The parameter used to describe the rate of diffusion in tissues is called the diffusion coefficient. In practice other sources of motion are present, such as the microcirculation. However, when strong gradients are applied this effect is minimal and so the term **apparent diffusion coefficient** or **ADC** is commonly used. Tissues in which diffusion is free have a high ADC, whereas those with restricted diffusion have a low ADC (Figure 25.1; Table 25.1).

Table 25.1 Equations of DWI.

	ADC (x10^{-3}mm^2/s)	relative signal when b=1000
Cerebral spinal fluid	2.94	0.05
Grey matter	0.76	0.47
White matter	0.45	0.63

Diffusion weighted images (DWI) are acquired by sensitizing this motion with the use of strong gradients. Two equal gradients are usually applied on either side of a 180° RF in a spin echo type sequence (called a **Stejskal Tanner scheme**). The gradient pulses are designed to cancel each other out if spins do not move, while moving spins experience phase shift. Signal attenuation therefore occurs in normal tissues with free random motion (high ADC) and high signal appears in tissues with restricted diffusion (low ADC). The amount of attenuation depends on the amplitude and the direction of the applied diffusion gradients and the ADC of the tissue (Table 25.2). Diffusion gradients applied in the X, Y and Z axes (see Chapter 27) are combined to produce a diffusion weighted image (isotropic image). When the diffusion gradients are applied in only one direction, signal changes reflect the direction of axons (anisotropic image).

Table 25.2 Typical ADC values.

Equations (if you like them)		
b= γ^2xG^{2}xδ^2x($\Delta-\delta/3$)	b is the b value or b factor (s/mm^2) γ is the gyromagnetic ratio (MHz/T) G is the gradient amplitude (mT/m) δ is the gradient duration (ms) Δ is the time between two pulses (ms)	The b value or b factor is a function of the amplitude, duration and interval of the gradients in the Skejskal Tanner scheme.

Diffusion gradients must be strong to achieve enough diffusion weighting. Diffusion sensitivity is controlled by a parameter 'b' that determines the diffusion attenuation by modification of the duration and amplitude of the diffusion gradient; 'b' is expressed in units of s/mm^2. Typical 'b' values range from 500 s/mm^2 to 1000 s/mm^2. As 'b' increases, diffusion weighting also increases and vice versa. The 'b' value is an extrinsic contrast parameter that controls how contrast is derived in a diffusion weighted image, in that high 'b' values exaggerate the differences in a tissue's ADC values (an intrinsic contrast parameter; see Chapter 6).

Clinical applications

DWI is commonly used in the diagnosis of stroke where areas of decreased diffusion, which represent infarction, are bright (Figure 25.2). In early stroke, cells swell and absorb water from the extracellular space and diffusion is restricted. These changes are seen very shortly after the stroke and are helpful to visualize the locality and extent of an infarct before other modalities are able to visualize them. DWI is also useful in other areas such as the liver, prostate and breast to differentiate between malignant and benign lesions and to differentiate solid from cystic areas. Very strong multidirectional gradients may be used to map white matter tracts, which have a lower ADC than surrounding grey matter. This technique is called diffusion tensor imaging or DTI (Figure 25.3). Other structures that contain fibres, such as muscle, may also be seen with this technique. Examples include skeletal muscle and the left ventricle.

Perfusion imaging

Perfusion is a measure of the quality of vascular supply to a tissue. Since vascular supply and metabolism are usually related, perfusion can also be used to measure tissue activity. Perfusion imaging utilizes a bolus injection of gadolinium administered intravenously during ultrafast T2* acquisitions. The contrast agent causes transient decreases in T2* in and around the microvasculature perfused with contrast. After data acquisition, a signal decay curve can be used to ascertain blood volume, transit time and measurement of perfusion. This curve is known as a time intensity curve. Time intensity curves for multiple images acquired during and after injection are combined to generate a cerebral blood volume (CBV) map. Mean transit times (MTT) of contrast through an organ or tissue can also be calculated.

Clinical applications

Perfusion imaging is commonly used in evaluation of ischaemic disease or metabolism. On the CBV map, areas of low perfusion (e.g. stroke) appear dark, whereas areas of higher perfusion (e.g. malignancy) appear bright (Figure 25.4).

The key points of this chapter are summarized in Table 25.3.

Table 25.3 Key points.

Things to remember:
DWI is a technique that sensitizes a spin echo type sequence to diffusion motion by using strong gradients.
The ADC is an intrinsic contrast parameter and signifies the net displacement of molecules in the extra-cellular space per second.
The b value is an extrinsic contrast parameter that controls how much the intrinsic ADC influences image contrast – hence the term diffusion weighted imaging.
Perfusion imaging involves rapidly imaging before, during and after injection of gadolinium to measure the perfusion kinetics of tissue.
Tissue contrast is determined by how quickly gadolinium changes the susceptibility of tissue as it first passes through the capillary bed.

Access Animation 12.1 relating to this chapter at www.westbrookmriinpractice.com/animations.asp

26 Functional imaging techniques

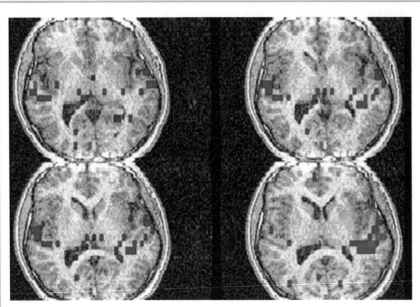

Figure 26.1 BOLD images of the brain. Functional areas in red.

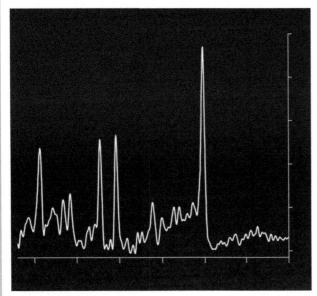

Figure 26.2 MR spectra of the brain.

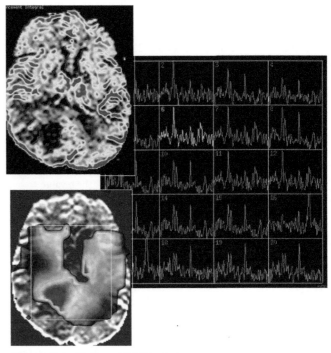

Figure 26.3 Multivoxel MRS technique.

F unctional imaging techniques are a group of protocols that visualize function as opposed to structural or anatomical detail.

Functional MR imaging (fMRI)

This is a rapid MR imaging technique that acquires images of the brain during activity or stimulus and at rest. The two sets of images are then subtracted, demonstrating functional brain activity as the result of increased blood flow to the activated cortex.

BOLD imaging

The most important physiological effect that produces MR signal intensity changes between stimulus and rest is called **blood oxygenation level dependent** or **BOLD**. BOLD exploits differences in the magnetic susceptibility of oxyhaemoglobin and deoxyhaemoglobin.

- **Haemoglobin** is a molecule that contains iron and transports oxygen in the vascular system, as oxygen binds directly to iron.
- **Oxyhaemoglobin** is a diamagnetic molecule in which the magnetic properties of iron are largely suppressed (see Chapter 1).
- **Deoxyhaemoglobin** is a paramagnetic molecule that creates an inhomogeneous magnetic field in its immediate vicinity that increases $T2^*$ (see Chapter 1).

At rest, tissues use a substantial fraction of the blood flowing through the capillaries, so venous blood contains an almost equal mix of oxyhaemoglobin and deoxyhaemoglobin. During exercise, however, when metabolism is increased, more oxygen is needed and hence more is extracted from the capillaries. The brain is very sensitive to low concentrations of oxyhaemoglobin and therefore the cerebral vascular system increases blood flow to the activated area. This causes a drop in deoxyhaemoglobin that results in a decrease in dephasing and a corresponding increase in signal intensity. Blood oxygenation increases during brain activity, and specific locations of the cerebral cortex are activated during specific tasks. For example, seeing activates the visual cortex, hearing the auditory cortex, finger tapping the motor cortex (Figure 26.1). More sophisticated tasks, including maze paradigms and other thought-provoking tasks, stimulate other brain cortices.

BOLD effects are very short lived and therefore require extremely rapid sequences such as EPI or fast gradient echo. The images are usually acquired with a long TE (40–70 ms) using echo-shifting techniques (see Chapter 22) while the task is modulated on and off. The 'off' images are then subtracted from the 'on' images and a more sophisticated statistical analysis is performed. Regions that were activated above some threshold level are overlaid onto anatomical images.

Clinical applications

The clinical applications are primarily in development of the understanding of brain function, including evaluation of stroke, epilepsy, pain and behavioural problems.

Spectroscopy

Spectroscopy provides a frequency spectrum of a given tissue based on the molecular and chemical structures of that tissue (Figure 26.2). Peak size and placement within the measured spectrum provide information on how an atom is bonded to a molecule. Most clinical spectroscopy looks at hydrogen, but advanced forms are able to evaluate other MR active nuclei. Spatial localization can be achieved by using the **stimulated-echo acquisition mode** or **STEAM**. The localized volume is generated via stimulated echoes from spins excited by three 90° RF pulses, and the conventional STEAM sequence detects the stimulated echo. A slice selective RF pulse is applied in conjunction with an X magnetic field gradient. This excites spins in an YZ plane. A 180° slice selective RF pulse is applied in conjunction with a Y magnetic field gradient. This rotates spins located in an XZ plane. A second 180° slice selective RF pulse is applied in conjunction with a Z magnetic field gradient. The second 180° pulse excites spins in a XY plane. The second echo is recorded as the signal. This echo represents the signal from those spins in the intersection of the three planes. Fourier transformation of the echo produces a spectrum of the spins located at the intersection of the three planes.

Clinical applications

Spectroscopy is now becoming a routine part of clinical imaging to evaluate tissue metabolism and identify tumour types (Figure 26.3).

The key points of this chapter are summarized in Table 26.1.

Table 26.1 Key points.

Things to remember:
Functional imaging techniques are used to image the function or physiology of a system rather than its anatomy.
fMRI relies on a process called BOLD to produce a signal in areas of the brain where there is increased activity after performing a function (such as finger tapping).
Spectroscopy is a technique that enables evaluation of tissue metabolism by looking at its molecular and chemical structures.

27 Gradient functions

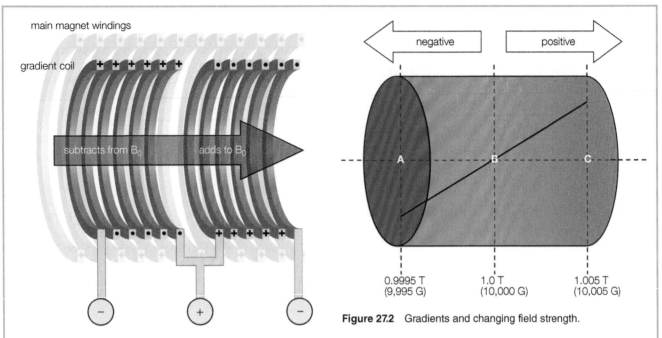

Figure 27.1   A gradient coil.

Figure 27.2   Gradients and changing field strength.

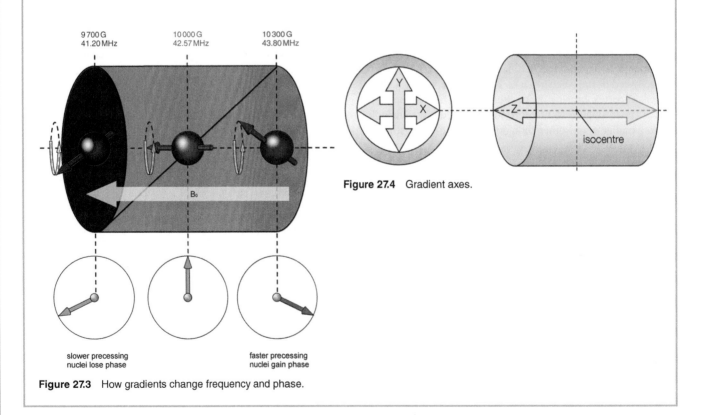

Figure 27.3   How gradients change frequency and phase.

Figure 27.4   Gradient axes.

MRI at a Glance, Third Edition. Catherine Westbrook. © 2016 John Wiley & Sons, Ltd. Published 2016 by John Wiley & Sons, Ltd.
Companion website: www.ataglanceseries.com/mri

Gradients are coils of wire that, when a current is passed through them, alter the magnetic field strength of the magnet in a controlled and predictable way. They add to or subtract from the existing field in a linear fashion so that the magnetic field strength at any point along the gradient is known (Figure 27.1). When a gradient is applied the following occur.

At **magnetic isocentre** (the centre of all three gradients), the field strength remains unchanged even when the gradient is switched on. At a certain distance away from isocentre, the field strength either increases or decreases. The magnitude of the change depends on the distance from isocentre and the strength of the gradient (Figure 27.2).

The slope of the gradient signifies the rate of change of the magnetic field strength along its length. The strength or *amplitude* of the gradient is determined by *how much current* is applied to the gradient coil. Larger currents create steeper gradients, so that the change in field strength over distance is greater. The reverse is true of smaller currents.

The polarity of the gradient determines which end of the gradient produces a higher field strength than isocentre (positive) and which a lower field strength than isocentre (negative). The *polarity* of the gradient is determined by the *direction of the current* flowing through the coil. As coils are circular, current either flows clockwise or anticlockwise.

The *maximum amplitude* of the gradient determines the maximum achievable *resolution*. Therefore, if at least one (and sometimes all three) gradients are steep, small voxels are achieved.

The *maximum speeds* at which gradients can be switched on and off are called the **rise time** and **slew rate**. Both of these factors determine the maximum scan speeds of a system (see Chapter 53). Therefore in fast sequencing the gradients have high slew rates.

How gradients work

The precessional frequency of the magnetic moments of nuclei is proportional to the magnetic field strength experienced by them (as stated by the Larmor equation; see Chapter 4). The frequency of signal received from the patient can be changed according to its position along the gradient. The precessional phase is also affected, as faster magnetic moments gain phase compared with their slower neighbours.

Imposing a gradient magnetic field therefore:
• changes the field strength in a linear fashion across a distance in the patient;
• changes the precessional **frequency** of magnetic moments of nuclei in a linear fashion across a distance in the patient (Table 27.1);

Table 27.1 Frequency changes along a linear gradient.

Position along gradient	Field strength (gauss)	Larmor frequency (MHz)
isocentre	10000	42.5700
1 cm negative from isocentre	9999	42.5657
2 cm negative from isocentre	9998	42.5614
1 cm positive from isocentre	10001	42.5742
2 cm positive from isocentre	10002	42.5785
10 cm negative from isocentre	9990	42.5274

• changes the precessional **phase** of magnetic moments of nuclei in a linear fashion across a distance in the patient (Figure 27.3).

These characteristics can be used to **encode** the MR signal in three dimensions. In order to do this there must be three orthogonal sets of gradients situated within the bore of the magnet. They are named according to the axis along which they work:
• The *Z gradient* alters the magnetic field strength along the *Z axis.*
• The *Y gradient* alters the magnetic field strength along the *Y axis.*
• The *X gradient* alters the magnetic field strength along the *X axis.*
• The **magnetic isocentre** is the centre of all three gradients. The field strength here does not change even when a gradient is applied (Figure 27.4).

There are only three gradients, but they are used to perform many important functions during a pulse sequence. For example, in gradient echo sequences, a gradient is used to refocus spins and produce a gradient echo (see Chapter 17). One of these functions is **spatial encoding**; that is, spatially locating a signal in three dimensions. In order to do this, three separate functions are necessary. Usually each gradient performs one of the following tasks. The gradient used for each task depends on the plane of the scan and on which gradient the operator selects to perform frequency or phase encoding.
• **Slice selection** – locating a slice in the scan plane selected.
• Spatially locating signal along the short axis of the image. This is called **phase encoding**.
• Spatially locating signal along the long axis of the image. This is called **frequency encoding** (Table 27.2).

Table 27.2 Gradient axes in orthogonal imaging.

	Slice selection	Phase encoding	Frequency encoding
Sagittal	X	Y	Z
Axial (body)	Z	Y	X
Axial (head)	Z	X	Y
Coronal	Y	X	Z
(Where X is across the bore of the magnet from right to left)			

The key points of this chapter are summarized in Table 27.3.

Table 27.3 Key points.

Things to remember:

When a moving current is passed through a conductor, a magnetic field is induced around it.

Gradient coils are conductors that cause a linear change in magnetic field strength along their axes when a current is passed through them.

The amount of current passing through the coil determines the amplitude, strength or slope of the gradient.

The direction of the current passing through the coil determines its polarity.

When a gradient is switched on it causes a linear change in magnetic field strength and therefore precessional frequency and phase of the magnetic moments of spins that lie along it.

Access the MCQs relating to this chapter on the book's companion website at www.ataglanceseries.com/mri

28 Slice selection

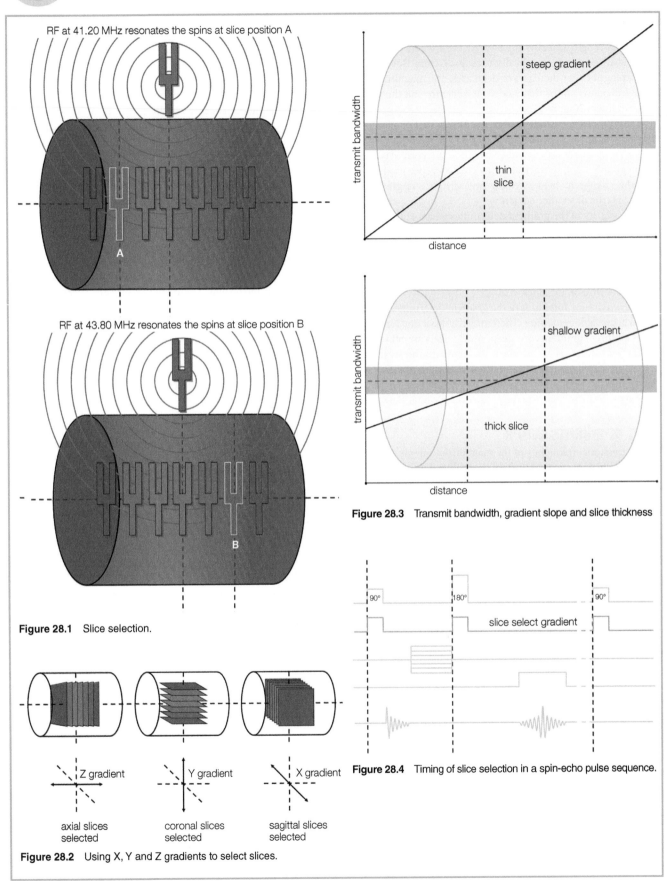

RF at 41.20 MHz resonates the spins at slice position A

RF at 43.80 MHz resonates the spins at slice position B

Figure 28.1 Slice selection.

Z gradient
axial slices selected

Y gradient
coronal slices selected

X gradient
sagittal slices selected

Figure 28.2 Using X, Y and Z gradients to select slices.

steep gradient

transmit bandwidth

thin slice

distance

shallow gradient

transmit bandwidth

thick slice

distance

Figure 28.3 Transmit bandwidth, gradient slope and slice thickness

90°   180°   90°

slice select gradient

Figure 28.4 Timing of slice selection in a spin-echo pulse sequence.

MRI at a Glance, Third Edition. Catherine Westbrook. © 2016 John Wiley & Sons, Ltd. Published 2016 by John Wiley & Sons, Ltd.
Companion website: www.ataglanceseries.com/mri

Mechanism

As a gradient alters the magnetic field strength of the magnet linearly, the magnetic moments of spins within a specific slice location along the gradient have a unique precessional frequency when the gradient is on (see Chapter 27). Transmitting RF at that unique precessional frequency therefore selectively excites a slice.

Example: a 1T field strength magnet with a gradient imposed that has changed the field strength between slices A and B causing a change in precessional frequency between slices A and B of 2.6 MHz (Figure 28.1).

- The precessional frequency of magnetic moments between slices A and B has changed by 2.6 MHz.
- To excite nuclei in slice A, an RF pulse of 41.20 MHz must be applied.
- Slice B and all other slices are not excited because their precessional frequencies are different due to the influence of the gradient.
- To excite slice B, another RF pulse with a frequency of 43.80 MHz must be applied. Nuclei in slice A do not resonate after the application of this pulse because they are spinning at a different frequency.

The scan plane selected determines which gradient performs slice selection. In a superconducting system the following usually apply (in an open magnet system, the Z and Y axes are transposed and some manufacturers transpose X and Y):

- The Z gradient selects axial slices, so that nuclei in the patient's head spin at a different frequency to those in the feet.
- The Y gradient selects coronal slices, so that nuclei at the back of the patient spin at a different frequency to those at the front.
- The X gradient selects sagittal slices, so that nuclei on the right-hand side of the patient spin at a different frequency to those on the left (Figure 28.2).
- A combination of any two gradients selects oblique slices.

Slice thickness

In order to attain slice thickness, a range of frequencies must be transmitted to produce resonance across the whole slice (and therefore to excite the whole slice). This range of frequencies is called a bandwidth and because RF is being transmitted at this instant, it is specifically called the **transmit bandwidth**.

The slice thickness is determined by the slope of the slice select gradient and the transmit bandwidth. It affects inplane spatial resolution and SNR (see Chapters 39 and 41; see Scan Tip 6).

- Thin slices require a steep slope or a narrow transmit bandwidth, and improve spatial resolution.
- Thick slices require a shallow slope or a broad transmit bandwidth, and decrease spatial resolution (Figure 28.3).

A slice is therefore excited by transmitting RF with a centre frequency corresponding to the middle of the slice, and a bandwidth and gradient slope according to the thickness of the slice required. The slice gap or skip is the space between slices. Too small a gap in relation to the slice thickness can lead to an artefact called **cross-talk**. This is caused because RF excitation pulses are Gaussian in shape (not exactly square). They have small 'tails' that overlap when RF pulses are too close together. This causes part of a slice to receive too much RF, resulting in cross-talk artefact (see Chapter 45).

The slice select gradient is always switched on during the delivery of the RF excitation pulse in the pulse sequence. It is switched on in the positive direction. The slice select gradient is also applied during the 180° pulse in spin echo sequences so that the RF rephasing pulse can be delivered specifically to the selected slice (Figure 28.4). Although not always shown, in all pulse sequences compensatory gradients are applied around each application of the slice select gradient. This is to compensate for the change of phase that the gradient imposes. This change of phase is not wanted in the slice selection process and is eliminated by these compensatory gradients.

The key points of this chapter are summarized in Table 28.1.

Table 28.1 Key points.

Things to remember:

Slices are selected by applying a gradient at the same time as the RF excitation and rephasing pulse.

The slice select gradient changes the magnetic field strength and therefore the precessional frequency of the magnetic moments of spins that lie along it.

An RF pulse at the specific frequency of magnetic moments of spins in a particular slice on the gradient causes resonance of the slice.

RF is transmitted width a bandwidth or range of frequencies on either side of the centre frequency of the slice.

Slice thickness is altered by changing either the slope of the slice select gradient or the transmit bandwidth.

Thin slices require either a steep slice select gradient slope or a narrow transmit bandwidth.

Thick slices require either a shallow slice select gradient slope or a broad transmit bandwidth.

Access Scan Tip 6 and the MCQs relating to this chapter on the book's companion website at www.ataglanceseries.com/mri

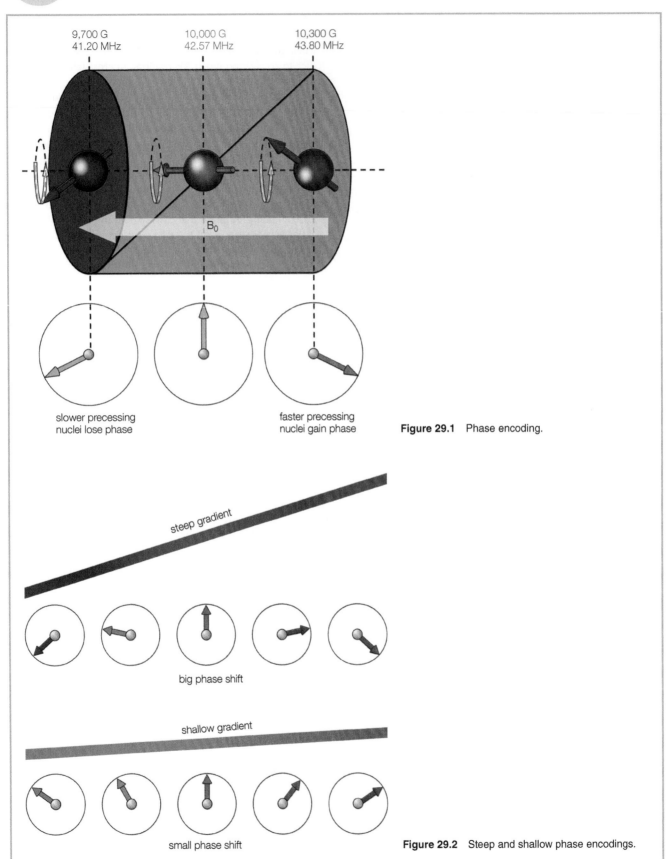

Figure 29.1 Phase encoding.

Figure 29.2 Steep and shallow phase encodings.

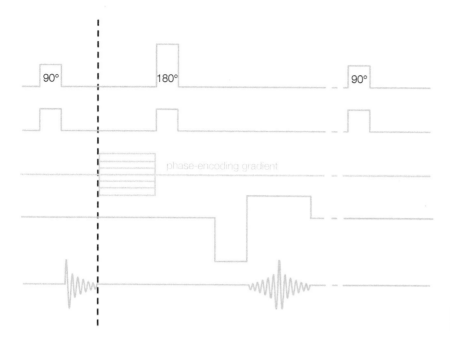

Figure 29.3 Timing of phase encoding in a spin echo pulse sequence.

After a slice has been selected and the slice select gradient switched off, the magnetic field strength experienced by spins within the excited slice equals the field strength of the system. The precessional frequency of the magnetic moments of spins within the slice is therefore equal to the Larmor frequency. The frequency of the signal from the slice also equals the Larmor frequency, regardless of the location of each signal within the slice. The system therefore has to use gradients to gain two-dimensional information representing the spatial location of the spins within the slice. When a gradient is switched on, the precessional frequency of the magnetic moment of a spin is determined by its physical location on the gradient.

Mechanism

The gradient changes the **phase** of the magnetic moment of each spin. The phase of a magnetic moment is its place on the circular precessional path at any moment in time (see Chapter 4). It can be compared with the position of a hand on a clock face.

The magnetic moment of a spin that experiences a higher magnetic field strength when the gradient is switched on gains phase relative to its position without the gradient on. This is because when the magnetic moment of a spin precesses at a higher frequency, it is travelling faster and therefore moves further around the 'clock' than it would have done with the gradient off.

If a spin experiences a lower magnetic field strength with the gradient on, its magnetic moment slows down relative to its speed or frequency with the gradient off, and loses phase.

Therefore, the presence of a gradient along one axis of the image causes a **phase shift** of nuclei along the length of the gradient (Figure 29.1). The degree of phase shift relative to isocentre depends on its distance from isocentre and the slope of the phase gradient.

When the phase-encoding gradient is switched off, the magnet moments of the spins return to the Larmor frequency but their phase shift remains; that is, they all travel at the same speed around the clock, but their positions on the clock are different. This phase shift is used to spatially locate the nuclei (and therefore signal) along one dimension of the image.

The slope or amplitude of the phase-encoding gradient determines the degree of phase shift. Steeper gradients produce a greater phase shift between two points than shallower gradients

(Figure 29.2). Steeper gradients increase the phase **spatial resolution** (see Chapter 41), the resolution of the image along the phase axis.

In most pulse sequences, the phase-encoding gradient is switched on after the RF excitation pulse has been switched off, and the amplitude and polarity of the gradient are altered for each phase-encoding step in standard sequences (see Chapter 32 and Figure 29.3). The number of times the phase-encoding gradient is switched on to a different amplitude determines the phase matrix (see Chapter 35).

This gradient is normally applied along the shortest axis of the anatomy, but is sometimes swapped to the longest axis (see Scan Tip 2). Unlike the slice select and frequency-encoding gradients, there are no compensatory gradients applied around each application of the phase-encoding gradient. This is because it is necessary for the change of phase that the gradient imposes to remain in order to spatially locate signal along the phase-encoding axis of the image (see Chapter 36).

The key points of this chapter are summarized in Table 29.1.

Table 29.1 Key points.

Things to remember:

Slices are phase encoded by applying a gradient along one axis of the two-dimensional image (usually the shorter axis).

The phase-encoding gradient changes the magnetic field strength and therefore the precessional frequency and phase of the magnetic moments of spins that lie along it.

Once this change of phase has occurred, the phase-encoding gradient is switched off so that the magnetic moments of spins precess at Larmor again, but their phase change remains.

The magnetic moment of each spin therefore has a slightly different phase position to its neighbour along the gradient.

The phase-encoding gradient is altered during the sequence. The number of times it is applied to a different amplitude determines the phase matrix. Its steepest application determines phase resolution.

 Access Scan Tip 2 and the MCQs relating to this chapter on the book's companion website at **www.ataglanceseries.com/mri**

Frequency encoding

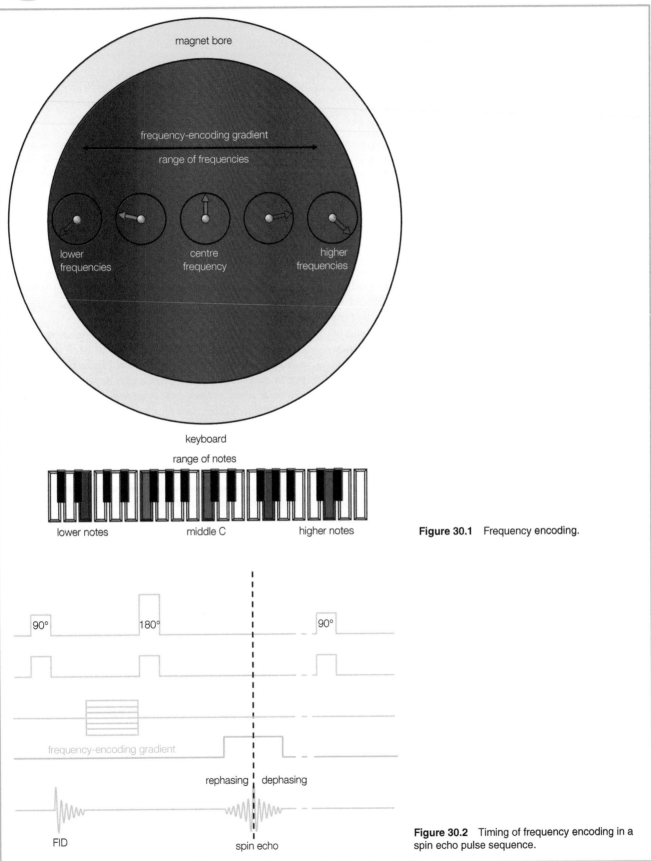

Figure 30.1 Frequency encoding.

Figure 30.2 Timing of frequency encoding in a spin echo pulse sequence.

MRI at a Glance, Third Edition. Catherine Westbrook. © 2016 John Wiley & Sons, Ltd. Published 2016 by John Wiley & Sons, Ltd.

Companion website: www.ataglanceseries.com/mri

After a slice has been selected and the slice select gradient switched off, the magnetic field strength experienced by spins within the excited slice equals the field strength of the system. The precessional frequency of the magnetic moments of spins within the slice is equal to the Larmor frequency. The frequency of the signal from the slice also equals the Larmor frequency, regardless of the location of each signal within the slice. The system has to use gradients to gain two-dimensional information representing the spatial location of the spins within the slice. When a gradient is switched on, the precessional frequency of the magnetic moment of a spin is determined by its physical location on the gradient. The change in frequency that this gradient produces is similar to the range of notes on a keyboard.

Mechanism

A gradient corresponding to the long axis dimension of anatomy in the image is usually switched on to locate signal along this axis, although this can be swapped (see Scan Tip 2). The frequency change caused by the gradient is used to locate each signal. It produces a frequency change or **frequency shift** in the following manner:

• The magnetic moments of spins experiencing a higher magnetic field strength due to the gradient speed up; that is, their precessional frequencies increase (similar to a high note on a musical keyboard).

• The magnetic moments of spins experiencing a lower magnetic field strength due to the presence of the gradient slow down; that is, their precessional frequencies decrease (similar to a low note on a musical keyboard; Figure 30.1).

This is called **frequency encoding** and results in a frequency shift of nuclei relative to their position on the gradient.

Frequency encoding allows the system to calculate where frequencies are located along an axis of the anatomy and the amplitude of each frequency. Every TR, data from this process is mapped into the horizontal axis of K space (see Chapter 31). Fourier mathematics is used to convert this frequency and amplitude data into separate pixels in the frequency direction of the field of view (FOV). The frequency data determines the pixel location. The amplitude data determines the signal intensity within the pixel.

Staying with the keyboard analogy, the spatial encoding process causes the creation of hundreds of different frequencies that are present in the echo. These frequencies have a variety of different amplitudes due to both extrinsic and intrinsic parameters (see Chapter 6). If the medium is sound as opposed to RF, the echo is analogous to a chord played by pressing hundreds of different keys at the same time. The amplitude translates to the loudness of each note. The Fourier process is a means of listening to this chord and mathematically calculating which keys were pressed, where they are located on the keyboard and how hard they were pressed.

The **frequency-encoding gradient** is switched on during the echo. It is often called the **readout** gradient because, during its application, frequencies within the signal are read by the system. The echo is usually centred to the middle of the gradient application and the readout gradient is usually switched on in the positive direction (see Chapter 32 and Figure 30.2). Although not always shown, in all pulse sequences a compensatory gradient is applied around each application of the frequency-encoding gradient. This is to compensate for the change of phase that the gradient imposes. This change of phase is not wanted in the frequency-encoding process and is eliminated by these compensatory gradients. Usually the compensatory gradient is a negative lobe applied before the positive readout lobe.

The *slope or amplitude* of the frequency-encoding gradient determines the *size of the FOV* in the frequency direction and therefore image resolution (see Chapter 41). The frequency-encoding gradient is usually applied along the longest axis of the anatomy, but can be swapped (see Scan Tip 2).

Did you know?

Each system has a minimum length of time required to switch all three gradients on and off. The speed with which it can do this depends on the sophistication of the gradients, their amplifiers and switching mechanisms. Steep gradients take longer to apply than shallow ones and an echo cannot be received until each gradient function has been performed. The selection of thin slices, high phase matrices or a small FOV requires each gradient to have a steep gradient slope. This results in the minimum TE increasing so that each of these gradients can be applied before the echo is read.

The key points of this chapter are summarized in Table 30.1.

Table 30.1 Key points.

Things to remember:

Slices are frequency encoded by applying a gradient along one axis of the two-dimensional image (usually the longer axis).

The frequency-encoding gradient changes the magnetic field strength and therefore the precessional frequency and phase of the magnetic moments of spins that lie along it.

The change of frequency is measured and enables the system to spatially encode signal in the frequency-encoding direction.

The amplitude of the frequency-encoding gradient determines the size of the FOV in the frequency-encoding axis. A small FOV requires a steep frequency-encoding gradient.

 Access Scan Tip 2 and the MCQs relating to this chapter on the book's companion website at www.ataglanceseries.com/mri

K space – what is it?

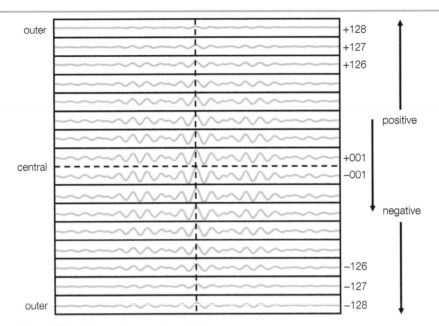

Figure 31.1 K space lines and numbering.

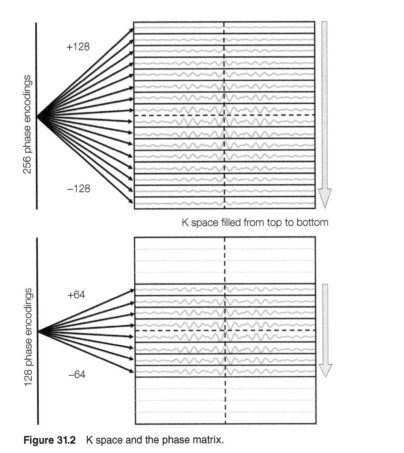

K space filled from top to bottom

Figure 31.2 K space and the phase matrix.

MRI at a Glance, Third Edition. Catherine Westbrook. © 2016 John Wiley & Sons, Ltd. Published 2016 by John Wiley & Sons, Ltd.
Companion website: www.ataglanceseries.com/mri

As a result of spatial encoding, spins are phase shifted along one axis of the image (see Chapter 29) and frequency shifted along the other (see Chapter 30). The system can now tell the individual spins apart by the number of times they pass across the receiver coil (frequency) and their position in the cycle as they do so (phase). However, in order to translate the information obtained from the encoding process into an image, the frequencies within the signal must be digitized through a process called **analogue to digital conversion** or **ADC** and stored as data points in an area of the array processor known as **K space**.

The image consists of a **field of view (FOV)** that relates to the amount of anatomy covered. The FOV can be square or rectangular, and is divided up into **pixels** or picture elements. The pixels exist within a two-dimensional grid or **image matrix** into which the system maps each individual signal. When the slice thickness is considered, a three-dimensional **voxel** is produced.

The number of pixels within the FOV depends on the number of frequency samples and phase encodings performed. Each pixel is allocated a signal intensity depending on the signal amplitude, with a distinct frequency and phase shift value. This is performed via by a mathematical process known as **Fast Fourier transform** or **FFT**. In its raw data form, the frequency of each signal is plotted against time; that is, the signal is measured in relation to its amplitude over a period of time. During FFT the system converts this raw data so that the signal amplitude is measured relative to its frequency. This enables the creation of an image, where each pixel is allocated a signal intensity corresponding to the amplitude of signal originating from anatomy at the position of each pixel in the matrix (see Chapter 29).

Before FFT can be performed, however, data points must be stored in K space. K space is a spatial frequency domain; that is, where information about the frequency of a signal and where it comes from in the patient is collected and stored. As frequency is defined as phase change per unit time and is measured in radians, the unit of K space is **radians/cm**. K space does not correspond to the image; that is, the top of K space does not correspond with the top of the image. K space is merely an area where data is stored until the scan is over.

Each slice has its own area of K space. For example, if 20 slices are selected there are 20 K space areas in the array processor.

K space is rectangular and has two axes:
- The **frequency axis** of K space is horizontal, centred in the middle of the K space perpendicular to the phase axis.
- The **phase axis** of K space is vertical, perpendicular to the frequency axis.

K space consists of a series of horizontal **lines**, the number of which corresponds to the number of phase encodings performed (**phase matrix**). Each line is filled with a series of data points, the number of which corresponds to the number of frequency samples taken (**frequency matrix**). Every time the frequencies in an echo are sampled, the data collected is stored as data points in a line of K space.

- The lines *nearest* to the centre are called the *central* lines.
- The lines *farthest* from centre are called the *outer* lines.
  The *top half* of K space is termed *positive*.
  The *bottom half* of K space is termed *negative*.

The polarity of the phase-encoding gradient determines whether the positive or negative half of K space is filled. Positive gradient slopes fill lines in the positive half of K space, and negative gradients fill lines in the negative half (see Chapter 37).

Lines are numbered relative to the central horizontal axis, starting from the centre (low numbers) and moving out towards the outer areas of K space (high numbers). Lines in the top half are labelled positive, those in the bottom half negative. The central lines of K space are always filled regardless of the phase matrix. For example, if a 128-phase matrix is required, lines +64 to −64 are filled rather than lines +128 to 0 (see Figures 31.1 and 31.2).

It is important to note that there is a centre line zero (0) that lies in the middle of the vertical axis of K space. When this line is filled with data, the phase-encoding gradient is not applied. This line is always filled so, when a 256-phase matrix is selected for example, 128 lines are filled in the top half of K space, followed by the zero line, followed by the bottom 127 lines (256 lines in total). This is commonly written as (+128, 0, −127). If the phase matrix is 128 then it is written as (+64, 0, −63).

K space lines are usually filled linearly; that is, either from top to bottom or from bottom to top (Figure 31.2). If filled from the bottom up then the above scenario of a 128-phase matrix is written as (−128, 0, +127)

K space is theoretically symmetrical about both axes; that is, data in the right-hand side of K space is identical to that on the left, and data in the top half is identical to that in the bottom half. This is called **conjugate symmetry**. However, in practice true symmetry only exists in the horizontal axis of K space. This is because motion artefact dominates in the vertical phase axis of K space, so symmetry of the data in this axis cannot be presumed (see Chapter 43).

The key points of this chapter are summarized in Table 31.1.

Table 31.1 Key points.

Things to remember:
K space stores information about where frequencies within the slice are located.
Data points acquired over time are laid out in K space during the scan and mathematically converted into information related to amplitude via FFT.
Every data point has information about the entire image locked inside it.

Access the MCQs relating to this chapter on the book's companion website at www.ataglanceseries .com/mri

32 K space – how is it filled?

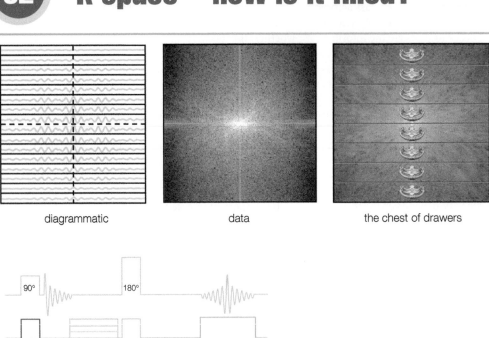

diagrammatic

data

the chest of drawers

Figure 32.1 K space – the chest of drawers.

slice select gradient chooses which chest of drawers

phase-encoding gradient chooses which drawer to open

frequency-encoding gradient chooses where to put the socks

Figure 32.2 K space filling in spin echo.

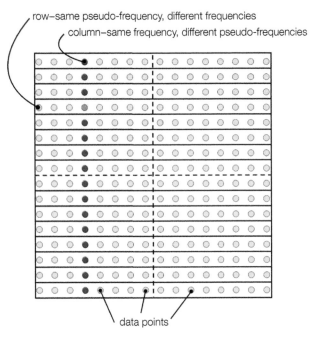

row–same pseudo-frequency, different frequencies

column–same frequency, different pseudo-frequencies

data points

Figure 32.3 Data points in K space.

MRI at a Glance, Third Edition. Catherine Westbrook. © 2016 John Wiley & Sons, Ltd. Published 2016 by John Wiley & Sons, Ltd.

Companion website: www.ataglanceseries.com/mri

The pulse sequence selected determines how K space is filled. Pulse sequences are defined as a series of RF pulses, gradient applications and intervening time periods. It is primarily the gradients that determine how K space is filled (see Chapter 37).

- The **slice select gradient** determines which slice is to be selected. As each slice has its own K space area, the slice select gradient determines which K space area is to be filled next (see Chapter 28).
- The **phase-encoding gradient** is the next gradient to be applied. The slope and polarity of this gradient determine which line of K space is to be filled. The polarity of this gradient determines whether a line in the top or bottom half of K space is filled (see Chapter 31). The slope of the phase gradient determines whether a central or outer line of K space is filled (see Chapter 33).
- The **frequency-encoding gradient** is switched on during the echo or signal. It is while this gradient is applied that frequencies from the echo are sampled, converted into data points and stored in each line of K space (see Chapter 34).

Did you know?

K space is analogous to a chest of drawers: just as a chest of drawers stores items such as socks in horizontal drawers, so K space stores data points in horizontal lines (Figure 32.1). Each K space area, and therefore each slice selected, represents a different chest of drawers.

Imagine that there is a pile containing nearly 2 million socks in the middle of a room surrounded by 30 chests of drawers, each containing 256 drawers. Your task is to place 256 socks into each drawer in every drawer of every chest of drawers. That would be quite a task, and to perform it efficiently you would have to fill each drawer methodically in a particular order. How do you think you could do this?

This is like the system computer having nearly 2 million data points from 30 slices (each slice having a phase and frequency matrix of 256) that it must place into 30 different K-space areas. Pulse sequences enable the system to perform this task methodically and efficiently. The gradients applied in a sequence determine how this may be done (see Chapter 37):

- The slice select gradient chooses which chest of drawers to walk up to (1–30).
- The phase-encoding gradient selects which drawer to open (1–256).
- The frequency-encoding gradient is on when 256 socks are put into this drawer from one side to the other (Figure 32.2).

This is why each gradient is applied in this order in a sequence, as it is obviously necessary to walk up to a chest of drawers first, then open a drawer and then place socks within the drawer.

Remember in this analogy that socks are data points and each chest of drawers represents a slice.

Once a particular drawer is filled, the *same* drawer in another chest of drawers is filled with socks. This requires the slice select gradient to be switched on again to excite another slice and hence walk up to another chest of drawers. The phase-encoding gradient must then be switched on again to the *same* slope and polarity to fill the *same* drawer in this chest of drawers. The frequency-encoding gradient is then switched on again so that 256 data points (socks) can be placed in the drawer.

This sequence is continued until the *same* drawer is filled in every chest of drawers (e.g. the top drawer of chests 1 to 30). When all the top drawers are filled in every chest of drawers, the TR period is repeated by applying another excitation pulse to the first slice. However, in this TR period a *different* drawer is filled to that in the first TR period. To do this the slope of the phase-encoding gradient is changed to open the next drawer down from the top. The sequence is continued, the same drawer being filled in each chest of drawers in a particular TR period. Every TR the slope of the phase gradient is changed to open the next drawer down, until all the drawers of all the chest of drawers are filled with socks (data points). The number of data points in each row or drawer corresponds to the frequency matrix selected. The number of data points in each column corresponds to the phase matrix and to the number of drawers in each chest of drawers (Figure 32.3). Using this example, there would be a total of 1,966,080 socks or data points stored ($256 \times 256 \times 30$).

This is only one way in which the drawers may be filled; there are many other permutations (see Chapters 36 and 38).

The key points of this chapter are summarized in Table 32.1.

Table 32.1 Key points.

Things to remember:
K space is analogous to a chest of drawers where the number of lines filled is the number of drawers in the chest of drawers.
Each gradient determines when and how the chest of drawers is filled.
In a standard sequence the same drawer is filled for each of the chests of drawers in a single TR period.
The number of drawers equals the phase matrix.
The number of socks or data points in each drawer equals the frequency matrix.

Access Animation 3.2 relating to this chapter at www.westbrookmriinpractice.com/animations.asp

K space and image quality

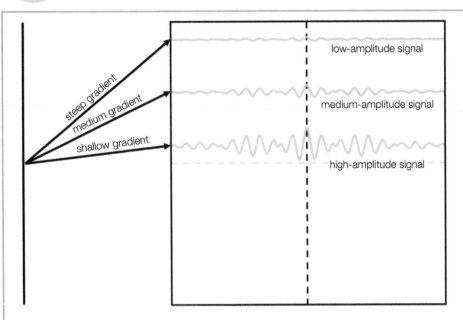

Figure 33.1 Phase gradient amplitude vs signal amplitude.

Figure 33.2 K space and signal and resolution data.

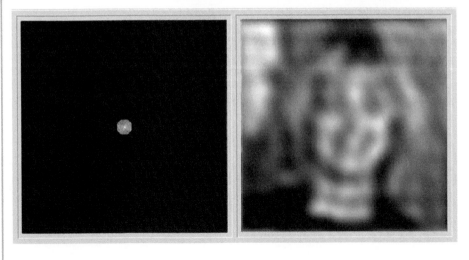

Figure 33.3 Image using central K space data points only.

MRI at a Glance, Third Edition. Catherine Westbrook. © 2016 John Wiley & Sons, Ltd. Published 2016 by John Wiley & Sons, Ltd.
Companion website: www.ataglanceseries.com/mri

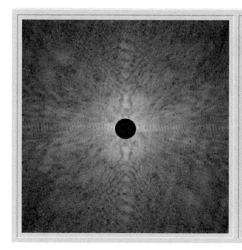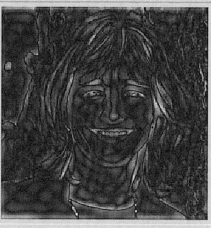

Figure 33.4 K space and signal and resolution data.

K space – signal and contrast

Phase data

The central lines of K space are filled with data produced after the application of shallow phase-encoding gradient slopes. The outer lines of K space are filled with data produced after the application of the steep phase-encoding gradient slopes. The lines in between the central and outer portions are filled with the intermediate phase-encoding slopes (see Chapter 31).

Shallow phase-encoding slopes do not produce a large phase shift along their axis. Therefore rephasing of magnetic moments by an RF pulse or a gradient is more efficient, as the inherent phase shift after phase encoding is small. The resultant signal therefore has a large amplitude, as a high proportion of the magnetic moments of spins are rephased by an RF pulse or a gradient to produce an echo.

Steep phase-encoding slopes produce a large phase shift along their axis. Therefore rephasing of magnetic moments is less efficient, because the inherent phase shift after phase encoding is great. The resultant signal has a small amplitude, as a small proportion of the magnetic moments of spins are rephased by an RF pulse or a gradient to produce an echo (Figure 33.1).

Therefore the central lines of K space, which are filled when shallow phase gradients are applied, contain data points that represent high signal amplitude and good contrast.

Frequency data

Frequencies sampled from the signal are mapped into K space relative to the frequency axis. The centre of the echo represents the maximum signal amplitude as all the magnetic moments are in phase at this point, whereas magnetic moments are either rephasing or dephasing on either side of the peak of the echo, and therefore the signal amplitude here is less. The amplitude of frequencies sampled is mapped relative to the central vertical axis, so that the centre of the echo is placed over this axis. The rephasing and dephasing portions of the echo are mapped to the left and the right and, as the echo is symmetrical about this axis, frequency profiles in the left half of K space are identical to those on the right (Figure 33.2).

Therefore the central points in K space contain data points that represent the highest signal amplitude both in terms of phase data and frequency data. Therefore if an image is produced solely from these data points, it has a high signal to noise ratio (see Chapters 39 and 40) and contrast. However, it also has poor resolution (Figure 33.3).

K space – spatial resolution

The outer lines of K space contain data produced after steep phase-encoding gradient slopes, and are only filled when many phase encodings have been performed. The number of phase encodings performed determines the number of pixels in the FOV along the phase-encoding axis. When a large number of phase encodings are performed, there are more pixels in the FOV along the phase axis and therefore each pixel is smaller. If the FOV is fixed, pixels of smaller dimensions result in an image with a high spatial resolution; that is, two points within the image can be distinguished more easily when the pixels are small (see Chapter 41). In addition, as the amplitude of the phase-encoding gradient slope increases, the degree of phase shift along the gradient also increases. Two points adjacent to each other have a different phase value and can therefore be differentiated from each other. So data collected after steep phase-encoding gradient slopes produces greater spatial resolution in the image than when using shallow phase-encoding slopes (see Scan Tip 8).

Thus the outer points in K space, particularly in the vertical axis, contain data points that represent the best resolution. If an image is produced solely from these data points, it has high spatial resolution (see Chapter 41). However, it also has poor signal and contrast (Figure 33.4).

The key points of this chapter are summarized in Table 33.1.

Table 33.1 Key points.

Things to remember:

The outer lines of K space contain data with high spatial resolution, as they are filled by steep phase-encoding gradient slopes.

The central lines of K space contain data with low spatial resolution, as they are filled by shallow phase-encoding gradient slopes.

The central portion of K space contains data that has high signal amplitude and low spatial resolution.

The outer portion of K space contains data that has high spatial resolution and low signal amplitude.

 Access Scan Tip 8 relating to this chapter on the book's companion website at **www.ataglanceseries .com/mri**

34 Data acquisition – frequency

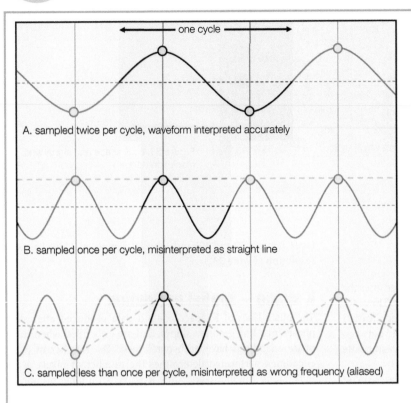

A. sampled twice per cycle, waveform interpreted accurately

B. sampled once per cycle, misinterpreted as straight line

C. sampled less than once per cycle, misinterpreted as wrong frequency (aliased)

Figure 34.1 The Nyquist theorem.

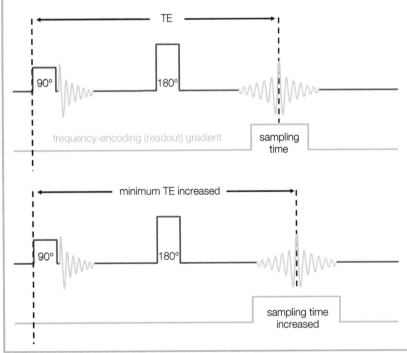

Figure 34.2 Sampling time and the TE.

The time available to the system to sample frequencies in the signal is called the **sampling time** or **sampling window**. It is the time for which the frequency encoding switches on. The rate at which frequencies are sampled during the sampling window is called the **digital sampling rate** or **frequency**. The digital sampling rate or frequency is determined by the receive bandwidth (the range of frequencies received). If the receive bandwidth is 32,000 Hz (or 32 kHz), this means that frequencies are sampled at a rate of 32,000 times per second.

The **Nyquist theorem** states that the digital sampling frequency must be at least twice the frequency of the highest frequency in the echo. If the digital sampling frequency obeys the Nyquist theorem then there are sufficient data points to accurately reproduce the original frequencies (Figure 34.1).

Enough data points must be collected to achieve the required frequency matrix with a particular receive bandwidth.

Changing the receive bandwidth

If the frequency matrix is 256, then 256 data points must be collected and laid out in each line of K space. The receive bandwidth (as determined by the digital sampling frequency) determines the number of times per second a data point is collected. The sampling time must be long enough to collect the required number of data points with the receive bandwidth selected.

For example, a receive bandwidth of 32,000 Hz is equivalent to a digital sampling frequency of 32,000 samples per second. This means that a data point is collected every 0.03125 ms. This is the sampling interval (1/32000 = 0.03125 ms).

If the frequency matrix is 256, then 256 data points must be collected during the sampling time or window. The length of this time period is therefore:

0.0325 × 256 = 8ms (Table 34.1)

If the receive bandwidth is reduced to 16,000 Hz, this is equivalent to a digital sampling frequency of 16,000 samples per second. This means that a data point is collected every 0.06125 ms. This is the sampling interval (1/16000 = 0.06125 ms).

However, only 128 data points can be collected at this rate in 8 ms (0.0625 × 128 = 8 ms). As the digital sampling frequency is not changed, the sampling time must be increased to collect the necessary 256 points. To acquire 256 data points the sampling time must therefore be doubled to 16 ms. This means that the frequency-encoding gradient must be switched on for 16 ms instead of 8 ms. As the echo is usually centred in the middle of the sampling window, the minimum TE increases as the sampling time increases (Figure 34.2).

Changing the frequency matrix

Using the previous example of a receive bandwidth of 32,000Hz, and a sampling window of 8 ms, let's see the effect of changing the frequency matrix from 256 to 512.

If the frequency matrix is increased without altering any other parameter, there are insufficient data points to produce a 512 frequency matrix in a sampling time of 8 ms. As the digital sampling frequency (as determined by the receive bandwidth) is not changed, the sampling time must be doubled to 16 ms to permit acquisition of 512 data points in each line of K space during the sampling window. As the echo is usually centred in the middle of the sampling window, the minimum TE increases as the sampling time increases.

Therefore either increasing the frequency matrix or reducing the receive bandwidth increases the minimum TE. These parameters have several important implications (see Scan Tips 3, 4 and 12).

The key points of this chapter are summarized in Table 34.2.

Access Scan Tips 3, 4 and 12 and the MCQs relating to this chapter on the book's companion website at www.ataglanceseries.com/mri

Access Animation 3.1 relating to this chapter at www.westbrookmriinpractice.com/animations.asp

Table 34.1 Equations of data acquisition.

Equations (if you like them)

$\omega_{sampling} = 2 \times \omega_{nyquist}$	$\omega_{sampling}$ is the digital sampling frequency (Hz) $\omega_{nyquist}$ is the Nyquist frequency (Hz), the highest frequency in the echo that can be sampled	If Nyquist is obeyed the highest frequency is sampled twice as fast as the Nyquist frequency and this determines the digital sampling frequency.
$RBW = 2 \times \omega_{nyquist}$ *therefore*	RBW is the receive bandwidth (Hz) $\omega_{nyquist}$ is the Nyquist frequency (Hz)	The receive bandwidth is the range of frequencies sampled on either side of the centre frequency. The RBW is therefore twice the highest frequency sampled.
$\omega_{sampling} = RBW$	$\omega_{sampling}$ is the digital sampling frequency (Hz) RBW is the receive bandwidth (Hz)	Combining the first two equations shows that when Nyquist is obeyed the receive bandwidth has the same numerical value as the digital sampling frequency.
$RBW = 1/\Delta Ts$	RBW is the receive bandwidth (Hz) ΔTs is the interval between each data point (ms)	The interval between each data point or sampling interval is determined by the receive bandwidth. If the sampling interval is short the receive bandwidth increases and vice versa.
$Ws = \Delta Ts \times M(f)$	Ws is the sampling window (ms) ΔTs is the sampling interval (ms) M(f) is the frequency matrix	The frequency matrix determines how many data points are collected in each line of K space. Therefore the sampling window is this number multiplied by the sampling interval.

Table 34.2 Key points.

Things to remember:

The sampling window is how long the system has to acquire the data. It is the time for which the frequency-encoding gradient is switched on.

The digital sampling frequency is how often the system samples frequencies during the sampling window. When Nyquist is obeyed this has the same numerical value as the receive bandwidth.

The frequency matrix determines how many data points must be collected during the sampling window.

The digital sampling frequency and the sampling window determine how many data points can be collected and therefore the frequency matrix.

If either the receive bandwidth or the frequency matrix isaltered, the sampling window is changed and this impacts on the TE, as the peak of the echo is positioned in the middle of the sampling window.

35 Data acquisition – phase

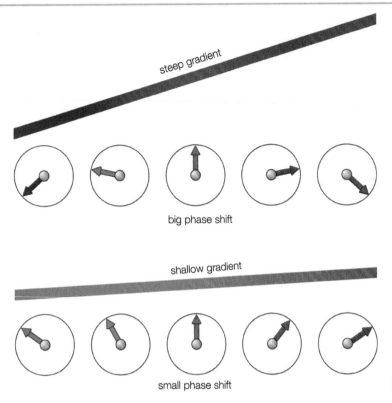

Figure 35.1 Phase-encoding slope and phase shift.

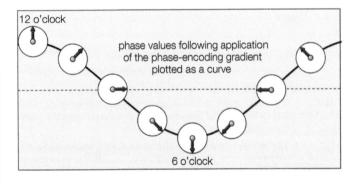

Figure 35.2 The phase curve.

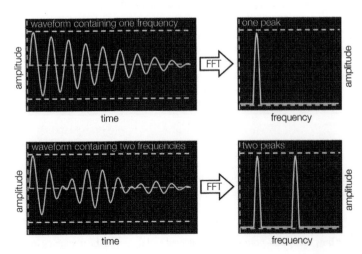

Figure 35.3 Fast Fourier transform.

MRI at a Glance, Third Edition. Catherine Westbrook. © 2016 John Wiley & Sons, Ltd. Published 2016 by John Wiley & Sons, Ltd.
Companion website: www.ataglanceseries.com/mri

A certain value of phase shift is obtained according to the slope of the phase-encoding gradient (see Chapter 29). The slope of the phase-encoding gradient determines which line of K space is filled with the data in each TR period. In order to fill different lines of K space, the slope of the phase-encoding gradient is altered after each TR. If the slope of the phase-encoding gradient is not altered, the same line of K space is filled all the time. In order to finish the scan or acquisition, all the selected lines of K space must be filled.

The slope of the phase-encoding gradient determines the magnitude of the phase shift between two points in the patient. *Steep* slopes produce a *large phase difference* between two points, whereas *shallow* slopes produce *small phase shifts* between the same two points (Figure 35.1). The system cannot measure phase directly; it can only measure frequency. The system therefore converts the phase shift into frequency by creating a waveform by combining all the phase values associated with a certain phase shift. This waveform or **phase curve** has a certain frequency that depends on the slope of the phase-encoding gradient (Figure 35.2).

In order to fill a different line of K space, a different phase curve must be obtained. If a different curve is not obtained, the same line of K space is filled over and over again. To create a different phase curve, a different phase shift is produced by the phase-encoding gradient. The phase-encoding gradient is therefore switched on to a different amplitude or slope, to produce a different phase shift value. Therefore, the change in phase shift created by the altered phase-encoding gradient slope results in a phase curve with a different frequency.

The frequency of this phase curve changes because the phase position of magnetic moments of spins within *each voxel* is altered differently when a different slope of phase-encoding gradient is applied. When the phase-encoding gradient is steep, the magnetic moments of spins in a voxel situated far away from isocentre are phase shifted further than when the phase-encoding gradient is shallow. If the pattern of this phase change is observed in a particular voxel *across the entire length of the scan*, another waveform is produced. The frequency of this is called a **pseudo-frequency.** Each voxel has its own pseudo-frequency depending on its location within the slice and so hundreds of different pseudo-frequencies are obtained, one for each voxel. These, along with frequencies obtained during frequency encoding, are sampled during readout. Each data point therefore has information about what happened during the spatial encoding process for the *entire slice.*

FFT is required to 'unlock' each data point and calculate the signal intensity for each voxel location (see Figure 35.3 and Chapter 31). This is achieved by calculating the amplitude of each spatial frequency (amplitude versus frequency information). The spatial frequency of each voxel is calculated from frequencies acquired as a result of frequency encoding and the pseudo-frequencies acquired as a result of phase encoding. This determines the spatial position of each voxel. The amplitude of each spatial frequency indicates the signal intensity of each voxel. A high-amplitude spatial frequency results in a high signal intensity in the voxel. A low-amplitude spatial frequency results in a low signal intensity in the voxel.

Did you know?

In order for the system to put data into different lines of K space every TR, the data has to change. There are potentially three ways of doing this:

- changing the slope of the slice select gradient every TR;
- changing the slope of the frequency-encoding gradient every TR;
- changing the slope of the phase-encoding gradient every TR.

The first two options change either the slice thickness (the slope of the slice select gradient changes this) or the size of the FOV in the frequency-encoding axis of the image (the slope of the frequency-encoding gradient changes this). Clearly these are parameters that need to stay the same every TR, so the only option is to change the phase-encoding gradient slope. This is the way the data is changed so that data is put into a new line of K space every TR.

The **NSA** is the number of TR periods for which the slope of the phase-encoding gradient remains the same (e.g. 2 × TR with the same slope of phase encoding = 2 NSA). In this example the slope of the phase-encoding gradient is the same for two successive TR periods before its slope is altered. Therefore twice the amount of data is placed into each line compared to 1 NSA, thereby improving the SNR but doubling the scan time (see Chapters 36 and 39).

The key points of this chapter are summarized in Table 35.1.

Table 35.1 Key points.

Things to remember:
The slope of the phase-encoding gradient is changed every TR (assuming 1 NSA). This changes the degree of phase shift across a certain distance in the patient.
Steep phase-encoding gradient slopes produce more phase shift than shallow ones.
The phase position of magnetic moments in voxels across the whole slice creates a waveform across the slice. This is called a phase curve.
The phase position of magnetic moments of spins within each voxel is altered differently when the slope of the phase-encoding gradient is altered and this is reflected by the production of a pseudo-frequency for each voxel. This is obtained by observing the change of phase shift of magnetic moments in a voxel during the entire scan.
Each voxel therefore has its own unique pseudo-frequency, so hundreds of pseudo-frequencies are obtained throughout the scan.
These pseudo-frequencies are sampled along with the frequencies obtained by frequency encoding and information from both processes is contained within a data point.
Each data point therefore has information about what happened during the spatial encoding process for the entire slice (not each voxel).
FFT is required to 'unlock' each data point and calculate the signal intensity for each voxel position in the slice.

Access the MCQs relating to this chapter on the book's companion website at **www.ataglanceseries.com/mri**

36 Data acquisition – scan time

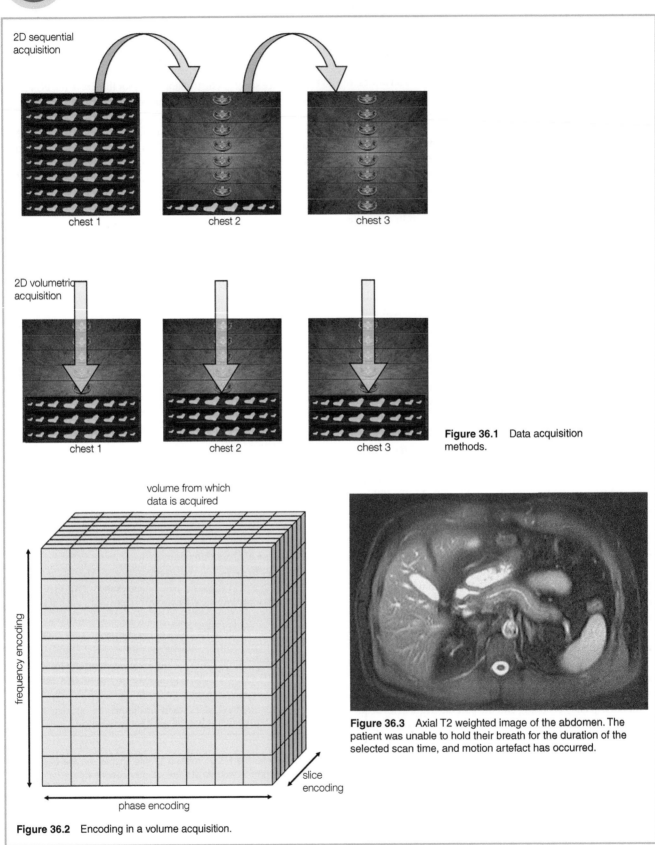

2D sequential acquisition

chest 1   chest 2   chest 3

2D volumetric acquisition

chest 1   chest 2   chest 3

Figure 36.1 Data acquisition methods.

volume from which data is acquired

frequency encoding

phase encoding

slice encoding

Figure 36.2 Encoding in a volume acquisition.

Figure 36.3 Axial T2 weighted image of the abdomen. The patient was unable to hold their breath for the duration of the selected scan time, and motion artefact has occurred.

The scan time is the time to fill K space. In 2D acquisitions it is a function of the following three parameters (Table 36.1).

TR

Every TR (assuming 1 NSA) the slope of the phase-encoding gradient is changed to fill a different line of K space for each slice. In the next TR period a different phase-encoding slope is applied to the slice to fill a different line of K space. The TR is therefore the time interval between filling a different line for each slice. So a long TR results in a longer scan time than a short TR because it takes longer to fill K space (see Scan Tip 10).

Phase matrix

The phase-encoding gradient slope is altered every TR (assuming 1 NSA) and is applied to each selected slice in order to phase encode it. After each phase encode a different line of K space is filled. The number of phase-encoding steps or lines of K space therefore affects the length of the scan. A high-phase matrix results in a longer scan time than using a low-phase matrix because more lines of K space are filled.

Number of signal averages (NSA)

The echo can be sampled more than once after the same slope of phase-encoding gradient. Doing so fills each line of K space more than once. The number of times each echo is sampled after the same slope of phase-encoding gradient is called the **number of signal averages (NSA)** or **the number of excitations (NEX)**. The higher the NSA, the more data that is stored in each line of K space. Note, however, that increasing the NSA increases the size or the amount of data in each data point, not the number of data points. Some of this data is signal, but some is noise. This is why increasing the NSA does not result in a proportional increase in SNR (see Chapter 39).

Types of acquisition

Two-dimensional sequential acquisitions acquire all the data from slice 1 and then go on to acquire all the data from slice 2, and so on. The slices are therefore displayed as they are acquired.

Two-dimensional volumetric acquisitions fill one line of K space for slice 1, and then go on to to fill the *same* line of K space for slice 2, and so on. When this line has been filled for all the slices, the next line of K space is filled for slices 1, 2, 3 etc. This is the type of acquisition discussed in Chapter 32 (Figure 36.1).

Three-dimensional volumetric acquisition (volume imaging) acquires data from an entire volume of tissue. The excitation pulse is not slice selective, and the whole prescribed imaging volume is excited. At the end of the acquisition the volume or slab is divided into discrete locations by the slice select gradient that, when switched on, separates the slices according to their phase value along the gradient. This process is called **slice encoding**. As slice encoding is similar to phase encoding, the number of slice locations increases the scan time proportionally, (see Scan Tip 6). Many thin slices can be obtained without a slice gap, thereby increasing resolution.

Reducing scan time

The longer a patient has to lie on the table, the more likely it is that he/she will move and ruin the image (Figure 36.3). To reduce scan times, the TR and/or the phase matrix and/or the NSA must be decreased. However, there are trade-offs associated with this (see Chapters 39, 41 and Appendix 1).

Reducing the TR to reduce scan time
- Reduces the SNR.
- Reduces the number of slices available in a single acquisition.
- Increases T1 weighting.

Reducing the phase matrix to reduce scan time
- Reduces phase resolution if the FOV remains unchanged.
- Increases the likelihood of truncation artefact.

Reducing the NSA to reduce scan time
- Reduces SNR.
- Increases some motion artefact.

There are some parameters that indirectly affect the scan time (see Scan Tips 3 and 4). Also note that in FSE or TSE the scan time is further reduced by using a longer ETL (see Table 36.1). In 3D imaging the scan time is further reduced by decreasing the number of slices.

The key points of this chapter are summarized in Table 36.2.

 Access Scan Tips 3, 4, 6 and 10 relating to this chapter on the book's companion website at www .ataglanceseries.com/mri

---

Table 36.1 Equations of scan time.

Equations (if you like them)		
in 2D imaging: $ST = TR \times M(p) \times NSA$	ST is the scan time (s) TR is the time to repeat (ms) M(p) is the phase matrix NSA is the number of signal averages	This equation shows how the scan time is calculated by the system.
in 2D TSE or FSE: $ST = TR \times M(p) \times NSA/ETL$	ST is the scan time (s) TR is the time to repeat (ms) M(p) is the phase matrix NSA is the number of signal averages ETL is the echo train length	The ETL determines how many lines of K space are filled per TR. The higher the ETL, the shorter the scan time.
in 3D imaging: $ST = TR \times M(p) \times NSA \times Ns$	ST is the scan time (s) TR is the time to repeat (ms) M(p) is the phase matrix NSA is the number of signal averages Ns is the number of slice locations	The number of slices in 3D imaging is equivalent to a slice matrix. This is why the scan time is multiplied by this number, as it is similar to the phase matrix.

Table 36.2 Key points.

Things to remember:
The scan time is always a function of the TR, phase matrix and NSA, because these parameters determine how long it takes to fill K space. In FSE and TSE sequences the scan time is decided by the echo train length or turbo factor, because multiple lines of K space are filled every TR. In 3D imaging the scan time is multiplied by the number of slice locations, because slices are located according to their phase position.

37 K space traversal and pulse sequences

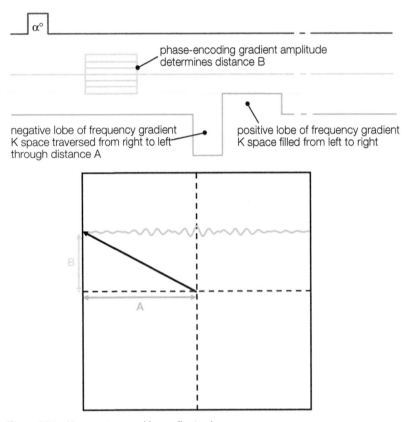

phase-encoding gradient amplitude
determines distance B

negative lobe of frequency gradient
K space traversed from right to left
through distance A

positive lobe of frequency gradient
K space filled from left to right

Figure 37.1 K space traversal in gradient echo.

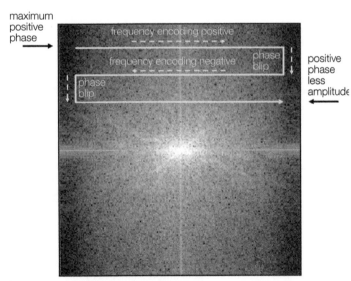

maximum
positive
phase

frequency encoding positive

frequency encoding negative

phase
blip

phase
blip

positive
phase
less
amplitude

Figure 37.2 Single-shot K space traversal.

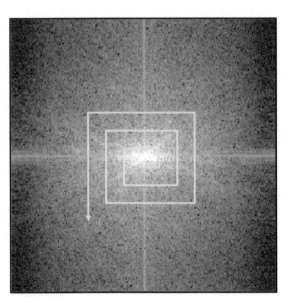

Figure 37.3 Spiral K space traversal.

MRI at a Glance, Third Edition. Catherine Westbrook. © 2016 John Wiley & Sons, Ltd. Published 2016 by John Wiley & Sons, Ltd.
Companion website: www.ataglanceseries.com/mri

The way in which K space is traversed and filled depends on a combination of the polarity and amplitude of both the frequency-encoding and phase-encoding gradients.

The amplitude of the *frequency*-encoding gradient determines how far to the *left and right* K space is traversed and this in turn determines the size of the FOV in the frequency direction of the image.

The amplitude of the *phase*-encoding gradient determines how far *up and down* a line of K space is filled and in turn determines the phase resolution. The maximum amplitude of phase encode that is applied – that is, the one that determines which lines are the outermost lines – affects the phase resolution or size of pixel on the phase direction.

The polarity of each gradient defines the direction travelled through K space as follows:
- *Frequency*-encoding gradient *positive*, K space traversed *from left to right*.
- *Frequency*-encoding gradient *negative*, K space traversed from *right to left*.
- *Phase*-encoding gradient *positive*, fills *top* half of K space.
- *Phase*-encoding gradient *negative*, fills *bottom* half of K space.

K space traversal in gradient echo

In a gradient echo sequence, the frequency-encoding gradient switches negatively to forcibly dephase the FID and then positively to rephase and produce a gradient echo (see Chapter 17).

When the frequency-encoding gradient is negative, K space is traversed from right to left. The starting point of K space filling is usually at the centre, as this is the effect the RF excitation pulse has on K space traversal. Therefore K space is initially traversed from the centre to the left, to a distance (A) that depends on the amplitude of the negative lobe of the frequency-encoding gradient (Figure 37.1).

The phase encode in this example is positive and therefore a line in the top half of K space is filled. The amplitude of this gradient determines the distance travelled (B). The larger the amplitude of the phase gradient, the higher up in K space the line that is filled with data from the echo. Therefore the combination of the phase gradient and the negative lobe of the frequency gradient determines at what point in K space data filling begins.

The frequency-encoding gradient is then switched positively and, during its application, data points are laid out in a line of K space. As the frequency-encoding gradient is positive, data points are placed in a line of K space from left to right. The distance travelled depends on the amplitude of the positive lobe of the gradient, which in turn determines the size of the FOV in the frequency direction of the image. If the phase gradient is negative, then a line in the bottom half of K space is filled in exactly the same manner.

K space traversal in spin echo

K space traversal in spin echo sequences is more complex, as the 180° RF pulse causes the point to which K space has been traversed to be flipped to the mirror point on the opposite side of K space, both left to right and top to bottom. Therefore, in spin echo, the frequency gradient configurations necessary to reach the left side of K space and begin data collection are two identical lobes on either side of the 180° RF pulse.

K space traversal in single shot

Filling K space in single-shot imaging involves rapidly switching the frequency-encoding gradient from positive to negative: positively to fill a line of K space from left to right and negatively to fill a line from right to left. As the frequency-encoding gradient switches its polarity so rapidly, it is said to oscillate.

The phase gradient also has to switch on and off rapidly. In the example shown in Figure 37.2, the first application of the phase gradient is maximum positive to fill the top line. The next application (to encode the next echo) is still positive, but its amplitude is slightly less, so that the next line down is filled. This process is repeated until the centre of K space is reached, when the phase gradient switches negatively to fill the bottom lines. The amplitude is gradually increased until maximum negative polarity is achieved, filling the bottom line of K space. This type of gradient switching is called **blipping**.

K space traversal in spiral imaging

A more complex type of K space traversal is spiral. In this example both the readout and the phase gradient switch their polarity rapidly and oscillate. In this spiral form of K space traversal, not only does the frequency-encoding gradient oscillate to fill lines from left to right and then right to left, but as K space filling begins at the centre, the phase gradient must also oscillate to fill a line in the top half followed by a line in the bottom half (Figure 37.3). This form of K space filling can be used in fast imaging techniques such as cardiac imaging.

The key points of this chapter are summarized in Table 37.1.

Table 37.1 Key points.
Things to remember:
The combination of RF pulses and gradients governs the type of pulse sequence, which in turn determines how K space is traversed.
The slice select gradient determines which area of K space is being traversed.
RF excitation pulses result in the system centering itself in the centre of K space.
RF rephasing pulses result in the point in K space to be flipped to the mirror point on the opposite side of K space.
The polarity of the phase-encoding gradient governs whether a line in the top or bottom half of K space is filled. Its amplitude controls which line is filled. In the image this determines the phase resolution.
The polarity frequency-encoding gradient governs whether K space is traversed from right to left or left to right. Its amplitude controls how far K space is traversed. In the image this determines the frequency FOV.

38 Alternative K space filling techniques

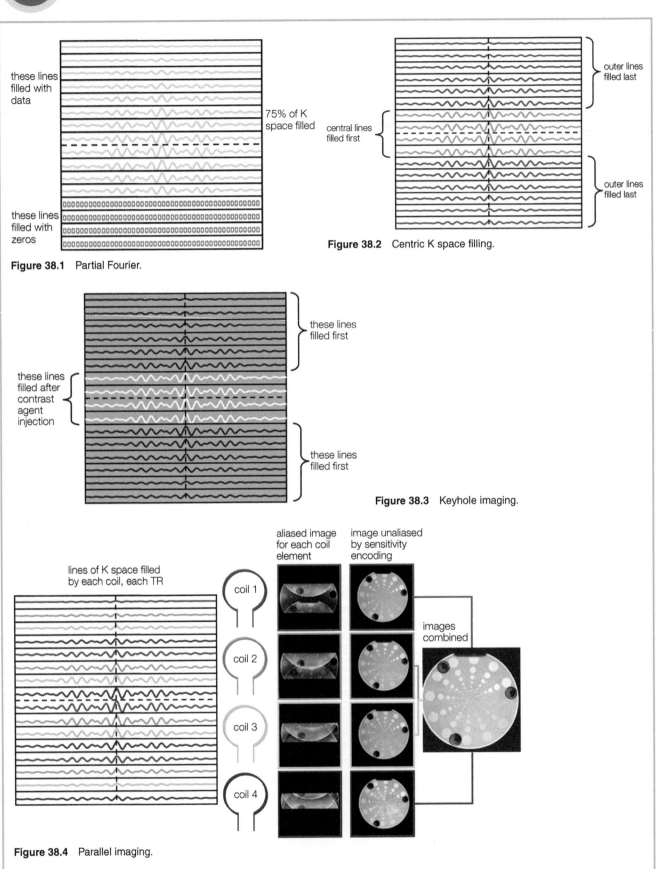

these lines filled with data

75% of K space filled

these lines filled with zeros

Figure 38.1 Partial Fourier.

outer lines filled last

central lines filled first

outer lines filled last

Figure 38.2 Centric K space filling.

these lines filled first

these lines filled after contrast agent injection

these lines filled first

Figure 38.3 Keyhole imaging.

lines of K space filled by each coil, each TR

aliased image for each coil element

image unaliased by sensitivity encoding

coil 1

coil 2

coil 3

coil 4

images combined

Figure 38.4 Parallel imaging.

MRI at a Glance, Third Edition. Catherine Westbrook. © 2016 John Wiley & Sons, Ltd. Published 2016 by John Wiley & Sons, Ltd.
Companion website: www.ataglanceseries.com/mri

Partial or fractional averaging

Partial averaging reduces the scan time because not all the lines are filled. As long as at least 60% of the lines of K space are filled during the acquisition, the system has enough data to produce an image. The scan time is reduced proportionally to the percentage of lines filled.

For example, if only 75% of K space is filled, only 75% of the phase encodings selected need to be performed to complete the scan, and the remaining lines are filled with zeros. The scan time is therefore reduced by 25%, but less data is acquired so the image has a lower SNR (see Chapter 39 and Figure 38.1).

Rectangular FOV

The incremental step between each line of K space is inversely proportional to the FOV in the phase direction as a percentage of the FOV in the frequency direction. In rectangular FOV the size of the incremental step between each line of K space is increased, and this therefore decreases the size of the phase FOV relative to frequency and a rectangular or asymmetric FOV results. As the incremental step between each line is increased, fewer lines are filled while maintaining the same K space area. As fewer lines are filled, the scan time decreases proportionally (see Chapter 41 and Scan Tips 8 and 13).

Anti-aliasing/over-sampling

The incremental step between each line of K space is inversely proportional to the FOV in the phase direction as a percentage of the FOV in the frequency direction. In anti-aliasing, the incremental step between each line is decreased and this therefore increases the size of the phase FOV relative to frequency. This means it is less likely that anatomy exists outside the larger FOV, thereby reducing aliasing. On some systems the extended FOV is discarded. On others it is maintained, thereby reducing spatial resolution.

As the incremental step between each line is reduced, more lines are filled while maintaining the same K space area. As a result over-sampling of data occurs, so there is less likelihood of phase duplication between anatomy outside the FOV and that inside the FOV in the phase direction. The scan time increases as more lines are filled. The NSA is either automatically reduced to maintain the original scan time, or some systems maintain the original NSA and the scan time increases proportionally (see Chapter 44 and Scan Tip 9).

Centric imaging

In this technique the central lines of K space are filled before the outer lines to maximize signal and contrast. This is important in sequences such as fast gradient echo where signal amplitude is compromised (see Chapter 24 and Figure 38.2).

Keyhole imaging

Keyhole techniques are often used in dynamic imaging after administration of gadolinium. The outer lines are filled before gadolinium arrives in the imaging volume. When it is in the area of interest, only the central lines are filled. Then data from both the outer lines and central lines are used to construct the image. In this way resolution is maintained but, as only the central lines are filled when gadolinium is in the imaging volume, temporal resolution is increased during this period. In addition, as the central lines are filled during this time, signal and contrast data are acquired, thereby enhancing the visualization of gadolinium (see Chapter 49 and Figure 38.3).

Parallel imaging

In this technique multiple receiver coils or channels are used during the sequence. Each coil or channel delivers data to its own unique lines of K space, and hence K space may be filled faster than if these coils are not used. For example, if two coils or channels are used, one coil supplies data to all the odd lines of K space and the other to all the even lines (see Chapter 52). During each TR period two lines are acquired together, one from coil 1 and the other from coil 2. Therefore the scan time is halved. The number of coils or channels is usually called the reduction factor and, unlike TSE (which also fills multiple lines of K space per TR), can be used with any type of sequence.

An image is produced for each coil. As each coil does not supply data to every line of K space, the incremental step between each line for each coil is increased. As a result, the FOV in the phase direction of each image is smaller than in the frequency direction and aliasing occurs. To remove the artefact, the system performs a calibration before each scan where it measures the signal intensity returned at certain distances away from each coil. This calibration or sensitivity profile is used to 'unwrap' each image. After this, the data from each image from each coil is combined to produce a single image. This technique allows considerably shorter scan times and/or improved resolution, for example phase resolution of 512 in a scan time associated with a 256-phase matrix (Figure 38.4).

The key points of this chapter are summarized in Table 38.1.

Table 38.1 Key points.

Things to remember:

The size of the incremental step between each line of K space is inversely proportional to the phase FOV size compared to frequency.

Rectangular or asymmetrical FOV is achieved by increasing the incremental step between each line. This is turn decreases the scan time, as fewer lines are filled.

Anti-aliasing is achieved by decreasing the incremental step between each line. This is turn increases the scan time, as more lines are filled. Data is over-sampled, so aliasing is less likely.

Partial averaging, keyhole and parallel imaging techniques are all used to reduce scan time, either by filling only part of K space (partial averaging and keyhole) or by using multiple coils to fill multiple lines per TR (parallel imaging).

 Access Scan Tips 8, 9 and 13 relating to this chapter on the book's companion website at www.ataglanceseries.com/mri

39 Signal to noise ratio

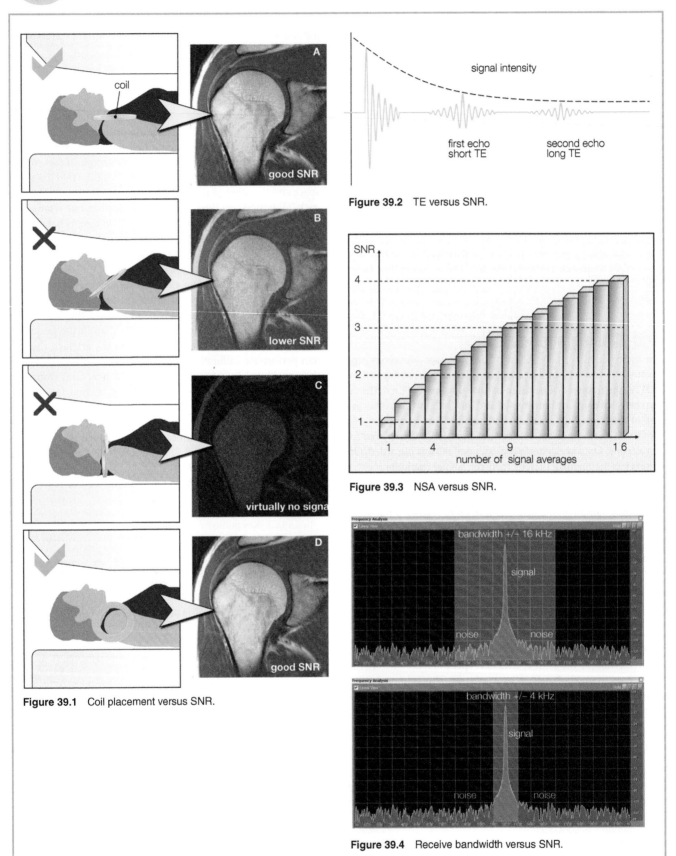

Figure 39.1 Coil placement versus SNR.

Figure 39.2 TE versus SNR.

Figure 39.3 NSA versus SNR.

Figure 39.4 Receive bandwidth versus SNR.

MRI at a Glance, Third Edition. Catherine Westbrook. © 2016 John Wiley & Sons, Ltd. Published 2016 by John Wiley & Sons, Ltd.
Companion website: www.ataglanceseries.com/mri

Signal to noise ratio (SNR) is defined as the ratio of the amplitude of the MR signal to the average amplitude of the background noise. The MR signal is the voltage induced in the receiver coil by the precession of the NMV in the transverse plane. It occurs at specific frequencies and time intervals (TE). Noise is the undesired signal resulting from the MR system, the environment and the patient. It occurs at all frequencies and randomly in time and space. To increase the SNR usually requires increasing the signal relative to the noise. There are several factors that affect the SNR (Appendix 1), of which the main ones are discussed here.

Proton density
Some structures contain tissues such as fat, muscle and bone that have a high proton density. On the other hand, the chest contains mainly air-filled lung spaces, vessels and very little dense tissue. When scanning areas with a low proton density, it is likely that measures to boost the SNR will be required.

Coil type and position
Small coils provide good local SNR but have a small coverage. Large coils provide much larger coverage but result in lower SNR. A good compromise is to utilize a phased array coil that uses multiple small coils that provide good SNR, and the data from these is combined to produce an image with good coverage (see Chapter 52).

The positioning of the receiver coil is also important. In order to receive maximum signal, receiver coils must be placed in the transverse plane perpendicular to the main field. In a superconducting system this means placing the coil over, under or to the side of the area being examined. Orientation of the coil perpendicular to the table results in zero signal generation (Figure 39.1).

TR
The TR determines how much the longitudinal magnetization recovers between excitation pulses and how much is available to be flipped into the transverse plane in the next TR period (see Chapter 8). Using a short TR, very little longitudinal magnetization recovers, so only a small amount of transverse magnetization is created, which therefore results in an image with poor SNR. Increasing the TR until all tissues have recovered their longitudinal magnetization improves the SNR, as more longitudinal magnetization (and therefore more transverse magnetization) is created. Although a short TR is required for T1 weighting, reducing this parameter too much may severely compromise the SNR.

TE
The TE determines how much dephasing of transverse magnetization occurs between the excitation pulse and the echo. When using a short TE, as very little transverse magnetization has dephased, the signal amplitude and therefore the SNR of the image are high. Increasing the TE reduces the SNR as more transverse magnetization dephases (Figure 39.2). Although a long TE is required for T2 weighting, increasing this parameter too much compromises the SNR (see Chapter 9).

Flip angle
The size of the flip angle determines how much of the longitudinal magnetization is converted into transverse magnetization by the excitation pulse. With a large flip angle all available longitudinal magnetization is converted into transverse magnetization, whereas with a small flip angle only a proportion of the longitudinal magnetization is converted into transverse magnetization. The flip angle is commonly varied in gradient echo sequences where a low flip angle is required for T2* and proton density weighted imaging (see Chapter 18). However, these also result in images with low SNR and hence measures may have to be taken to improve the flip angle.

Number of signal averages (NSA)
This parameter determines the number of times frequencies in the signal are sampled after the same slope of phase-encoding gradient (see Chapter 36). Increasing the NSA increases the signal collected. However, noise is also sampled. As noise occurs at all frequencies and randomly, doubling the NSA only increases the SNR by the square of root of 2 (Table 39.1). Because of this relationship, the benefits of increasing the SNR as the NSA increases are reduced, but the scan time increases proportionally (Figure 39.3).

Table 39.1 Equations of SNR.

Equations (if you like them)		
SNR α FOV SNR α 1/matrix SNR α S_t	S_t is slice thickness (mm)	These relationships show that the SNR is related to the voxel volume. SNR increases as FOV and slice thickness increase, but decreases if the matrix increases.
SNR α √NSA SNR α √1/RBW	The proportional sign is used in these relationships as there are many other factors that affect SNR such as TR, TE, flip angle and proton density.	These relationships show that the SNR is related to the amount of data in K space and that as the bandwidth decreases, SNR increases.

Receive bandwidth
This is the range of frequencies sampled during readout (see Chapter 34). Reducing the receive bandwidth reduces the proportion of noise sampled relative to signal (Figure 39.4). Reducing the receive bandwidth is a very effective way of boosting the SNR. However, reducing the bandwidth increases:
• the minimum TE, so this technique is not suitable for T1 or PD imaging (see Chapter 34);
• an artefact known as chemical shift (see Chapter 42).

Despite these trade-offs, reduced receive bandwidths should be used when a short TE is not required (T2 weighting) and when fat is not present (see Scanning Tips 4 and 5). An example is an examination when fat is suppressed in conjunction with T2 weighting, for instance T2 TSE and STIR (Figure 16.4).

The FOV, matrix and slice thickness also affect the SNR (see Chapter 41), as does the field strength (Table 39.1).

The key points of this chapter are summarized in Table 39.2.

Table 39.2 Key points.

Things to remember:
Signal amplitude is altered in several ways, including using a long TR, a short TE, a large flip angle and a good coil.
Noise is random and largely not alterable, although when using a narrow receive bandwidth fewer noise frequencies are sampled.
The SNR is therefore usually improved by increasing signal relative to noise rather than the other way round.
The trade-offs associated with improving SNR are summarized in Appendix 1.

 Access Scan Tips 4 and 5 and the MCQs relating to this chapter on the book's companion website at www.ataglanceseries.com/mri

40 Contrast to noise ratio

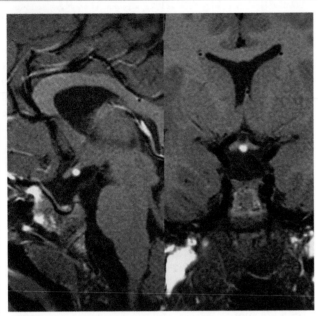

Figure 40.1 Sagittal (left) and coronal (right) T1 weighted image after contrast showing an ectopic posterior pituitary.

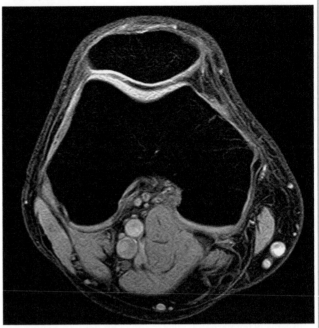

Figure 40.2 Axial slice of the knee from a 3D acquisition using chemical suppression.

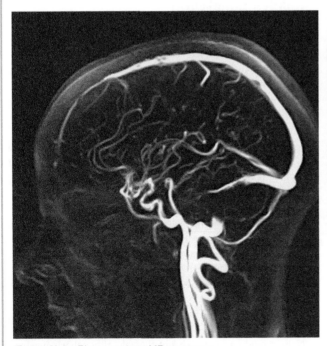

Figure 40.3 Phase contrast MR venogram.

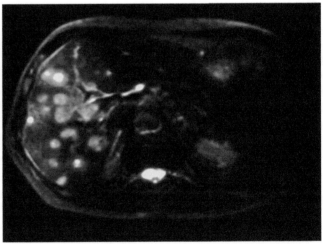

Figure 40.4 Axial T2 weighted image of the liver with chemical suppression. There is a good CNR between the liver lesions and normal liver using this technique, although the overall image quality is poor.

MRI at a Glance, Third Edition. Catherine Westbrook. © 2016 John Wiley & Sons, Ltd. Published 2016 by John Wiley & Sons, Ltd.
Companion website: www.ataglanceseries.com/mri

The **contrast to noise ratio** or **CNR** is defined as the difference in SNR between two adjacent areas. It is controlled by the same factors that affect SNR. The CNR is probably the most important image quality factor, as the objective of any examination is to produce an image where pathology is clearly seen relative to normal anatomy. Visualization of a lesion increases if the CNR between it and surrounding anatomy is high. The CNR is increased by the following.

Administration of contrast

Contrast agents such as gadolinium produce T1 shortening of lesions, especially those that cause a breakdown in the blood–brain barrier. As a result, enhancing tissue appears bright on T1 weighted images and therefore there is a good CNR between it and surrounding non-enhancing tissue (see Chapter 50 and Figure 40.1).

Magnetization transfer contrast

Magnetization transfer contrast (**MTC**) uses additional RF pulses to suppress hydrogen protons that are not free but bound to macromolecules and cell membranes. These pulses are either applied at a frequency away from the Larmor frequency, where they are known as **off resonant**, or nearer to the centre frequency, where they are known as **on resonant**. As a result of the application of these pulses, magnetization is transferred to the free protons suppressing the signal in certain types of tissue.

Chemical suppression techniques

These techniques are used to suppress signal from either fat or water or other substances such as silicone. They improve the CNR because the signal from unwanted tissue is removed. They are often used in conjunction with T2 weighting so that pathology has a high signal compared to the unwanted tissue (Figures 40.2 and 40.4). Fat is the commonest tissue to suppress. There are a variety of ways to do this based on the fact that fat and water either precess at different frequencies (chemical shift, see Chapter 42) or have a different relaxation time (see Chapter 7).

Chemical shift techniques include the Dixon technique, spectral fat suppression and water excitation.

The Dixon technique relies on the fact that due to the difference in precessional frequency between fat and water, their magnetic moments are sometimes in phase and sometimes out of phase (see Chapter 42). Two images are acquired: one with the spins in phase and one with them out of phase. Separate fat-only or water-only images are produced.

Spectral fat suppression relies on the fact that fat and water have different precessional frequencies at the same field strength.

An RF pulse at the frequency specifically of fat is applied to excite fat, but the transverse magnetization of fat is spoiled, leaving only water to produce an image.

In water excitation a binomial RF excitation pulse is applied that fully excites water but only minimally excites fat.

Techniques that rely on the difference in relation times of fat and water include STIR (see Chapter 16 and spectrally adiabatic inversion recovery or SPAIR). The fat spins are specifically inverted using an RF pulse with a frequency specifically of fat. Any transverse magnetization of fat is spoiled. The inversion time is selected to match the null point of fat, so there is no transverse component in fat when the echo is collected.

Flow techniques

These are used to provide images where flowing spins produce signal and other tissues do not. An example of this is phase contrast angiography (see Chapter 48). These techniques produce images where the CNR between flow and non-flow is very high and enables clear visualization of vessels (Figure 40.3).

T2 weighting

T2 weighting is specifically used to increase the CNR between normal and abnormal tissue. Pathology is often bright on a T2 weighted image as it contains water. As a result, pathology is more conspicuous than on T1 or PD weighted images.

Sometimes acquiring an image with good CNR means compromising other image quality factors. An example is in the liver when, in T1 weighted images, lesions and normal liver may be **isointense** (the same signal intensity). Fat-suppressed T2 weighted imaging with a very long TE produces an image where the CNR between lesions (bright) and normal liver (dark) is increased. However the SNR, spatial resolution and scan time are usually compromised in these images because of the parameters selected (Figure 40.4).

The key points of this chapter are summarized in Table 40.1.

Table 40.1 Key points.

Things to remember:

CNR is the difference in SNR between two adjacent areas.

It is important to maximize the CNR so that pathology is clearly seen as distinct from normal anatomy or so that one structure is clearly seen next to another.

CNR is improved by increasing the signal from pathology or structures that are important to see (e.g. positive contrast agents, T2 weighting, flow techniques).

CNR is improved by decreasing signal from normal structures (e.g. chemical suppression, MTC).

(41) **Spatial resolution**

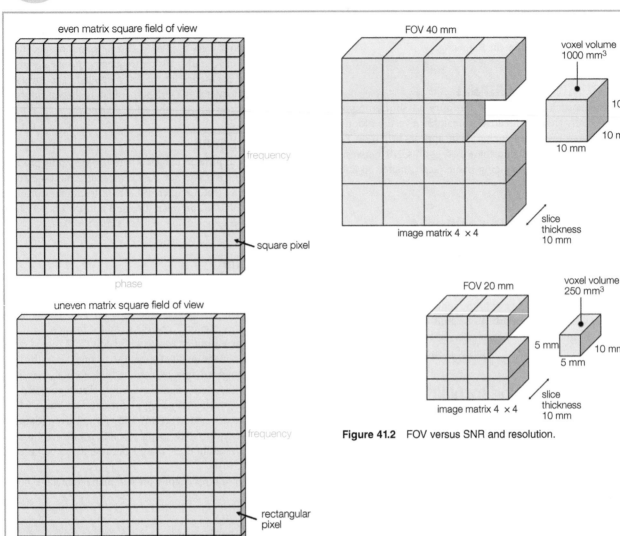

even matrix square field of view

frequency

square pixel

phase

uneven matrix square field of view

frequency

rectangular pixel

phase

Figure 41.1 Pixel size versus matrix size. Voxels are larger on the lower diagram, which results in a better SNR but poorer resolution than the upper diagram.

FOV 40 mm

voxel volume 1000 mm³

10 mm

10 mm

10 mm

image matrix 4 × 4

slice thickness 10 mm

FOV 20 mm

voxel volume 250 mm³

5 mm

10 mm

5 mm

image matrix 4 × 4

slice thickness 10 mm

Figure 41.2 FOV versus SNR and resolution.

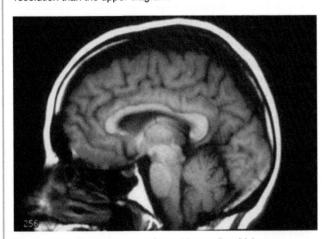

Figure 41.3 Sagittal image using a 10 mm slice thickness.

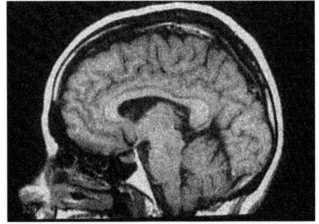

Figure 41.4 Sagittal image using a 3 mm slice thickness.

MRI at a Glance, Third Edition. Catherine Westbrook. © 2016 John Wiley & Sons, Ltd. Published 2016 by John Wiley & Sons, Ltd.

Companion website: www.ataglanceseries.com/mri

Spatial resolution is defined as the ability to distinguish between two points that are close together in the patient. It is entirely controlled by the size of the voxel.

The imaging volume is divided into slices.

- Each slice displays an area of anatomy defined as the **field of view or FOV**.
- The FOV is divided into pixels, the size of which is controlled by the **image matrix**.
- The **voxel** is defined as the pixel area multiplied by the slice thickness.

Therefore the factors that affect the voxel volume are:

- slice thickness;
- FOV;
- image matrix.

Voxel volume and SNR

The size of the voxel determines how much signal each voxel contains. Large voxels have higher signal than small ones because there are more spins in a large voxel to contribute to the signal. Therefore any setting of FOV, image matrix size or slice thickness that results in large voxels leads to a higher SNR per voxel. However, as the voxels increase in size, resolution decreases. There is thus a direct conflict between SNR and resolution in the geometry of the voxel.

Voxel volume and resolution

Small voxels improve resolution as they increase the likelihood of two points, close together in the patient, being in separate voxels and therefore distinguishable from each other. Changing any dimension of the voxel changes the resolution, but there is a direct trade-off with SNR (see Scan Tip 7 and Appendix 1).

Changing the matrix and SNR

This changes the dimension of each pixel along the frequency-encoding and phase-encoding axes, depending on whether just one or both matrices are altered. If there are fewer pixels to map over the FOV, each pixel is larger. The SNR of each voxel therefore increases. Changing the phase matrix also changes scan time (see Tables 36.1 and 39.1).

Changing the matrix and resolution

Changing the image matrix alters the number of pixels that fit into the FOV. Therefore, as the image matrix increases, pixel and thus voxel size decrease, assuming the FOV is unchanged. This increases resolution but reduces SNR. Changing the phase matrix also changes scan time (see Scan Tip 13 and Figure 41.1).

Changing the FOV and SNR

The pixel (and therefore voxel) dimensions along each axis of the FOV change as the FOV changes. The SNR of each voxel increases by a factor of 4, because the dimensions of each pixel double along each axis of the FOV (see Table 39.1).

Changing the FOV and resolution

In Figure 41.2 an FOV of 40 mm, a non-representative matrix of 4 × 4 and a slice thickness of 10 mm are illustrated. This produces a voxel volume of 1000 mm³. Halving the FOV to 20 mm reduces the voxel volume and therefore the SNR to a quarter of its original size, although spatial resolution is doubled along both the frequency and phase axes.

As reducing the FOV affects the size of the pixel along both axes, the voxel volume is significantly reduced. Decreasing the FOV therefore has a drastic effect on SNR. Using a small FOV is appropriate when using small coils that boost local SNR, but should be employed with caution when using a large coil, as SNR is severely compromised unless measures such as increasing the NSA are utilized.

Changing slice thickness and SNR

Changing the slice thickness changes the voxel volume along the dimension of the slice. Thick slices cover more of the patient's body tissue and therefore have more spinning protons within them. SNR thus increases in proportion to increase in slice thickness (see Scan Tip 6 and Table 39.1).

Changing slice thickness and resolution

Changing the slice thickness changes the voxel volume proportionally and results in a change in both SNR and resolution. In Figure 41.3 a thick slice of 10 mm has been used. This image has good SNR, but there is partial voluming leading to poor in-slice resolution. In Figure 41.4 the slice thickness has been reduced to 3 mm. This image has poorer SNR due to a smaller voxel volume, and the in-slice resolution has improved. However, as the pixel area has not changed, the image resolution is also unchanged.

The key points of this chapter are summarized in Table 41.1.

Table 41.1 Key points.

Things to remember:
Resolution is the ability to visualize two points that are close together in the patient as separate points in the image.
Resolution depends on voxels being small and is therefore achieved by using a small FOV, a thin slice and a high matrix.
Small voxels results in poor SNR.
The trade-offs associated with improving resolution are summarized in Appendix 1.

Access Scan Tips 6, 7 and 13 relating to this chapter on the book's companion website at www.ataglanceseries.com/mri

42 Chemical shift artefacts

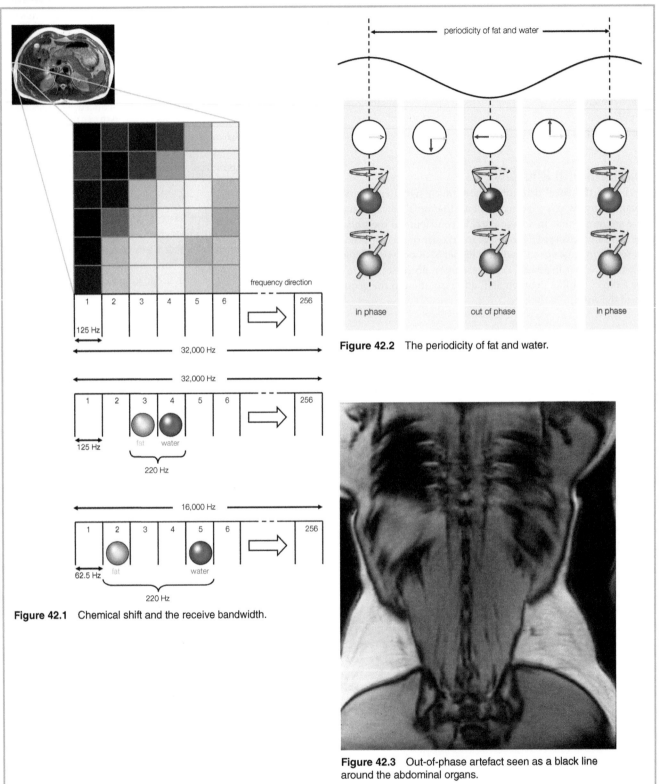

frequency direction

1 2 3 4 5 6 256

125 Hz

32,000 Hz

32,000 Hz

1 2 3 4 5 6 256

125 Hz

fat water

220 Hz

16,000 Hz

1 2 3 4 5 6 256

62.5 Hz

fat water

220 Hz

Figure 42.1 Chemical shift and the receive bandwidth.

periodicity of fat and water

in phase   out of phase   in phase

Figure 42.2 The periodicity of fat and water.

Figure 42.3 Out-of-phase artefact seen as a black line around the abdominal organs.

MRI at a Glance, Third Edition. Catherine Westbrook. © 2016 John Wiley & Sons, Ltd. Published 2016 by John Wiley & Sons, Ltd.
Companion website: www.ataglanceseries.com/mri

Fat and water naturally precess at slightly different frequencies at the same field strength. This is because hydrogen exists in a very different environment in these tissues (see Chapter 6). In water, hydrogen is linked to oxygen; in fat, it is linked to carbon. Due to the two different chemical environments, hydrogen in fat resonates at a lower frequency than in water. The difference in their precessional frequencies is called **chemical shift** and causes two artefacts.

Chemical shift artefact is displacement of signal between fat and water along the frequency axis of the image due to their different precessional frequencies. Its magnitude depends on the magnetic field strength of the system and significantly increases at higher field strengths. The **receive bandwidth** is one of the factors that controls chemical shift. It also controls SNR (see Chapter 39). The receive bandwidth determines the range of frequencies that must be mapped across pixels in the frequency direction of the FOV. It is selected to receive signal with frequencies slightly higher and lower than the centre frequency (see Chapter 34). It is usually measured in kHz (kilohertz). At 1.5 T with a receive bandwidth of ±16 kHz on either side of the centre frequency, each pixel contains a range of frequencies, for instance 125 Hz per pixel if the frequency matrix is 256, or 62.5 Hz per pixel if the frequency matrix is 512 (Table 42.1). If fat and water coexist in the same place in the patient, the frequency-encoding process maps fat hydrogen several Hz lower than water hydrogen into the image. They therefore appear in different pixels in the image, despite coexisting in the patient. As the receive bandwidth is reduced, fewer frequencies are mapped across the same number of pixels. As a result, chemical shift artefact increases see Figure 42.1 and Scan Tip 4).

Table 42.1 Equations of chemical shift.

Equations (if you like them)		
$\omega_{csf} = \omega_0 \times C_s$	ω_{csf} is the chemical shift frequency difference between fat and water (Hz) ω_0 is the precessional frequency (Hz) C_s is the chemical shift (3.5 ppm or 3.5×10^{-6})	At 1.5 T, for example, the precessional frequency is 63.86 MHz (63.86×10^6), therefore the chemical shift frequency difference between fat and water at 1.5 T is 220 Hz.
$CS_p = \dfrac{C_s \times \gamma \times B_0 \times FOV}{RBW/Matrix(f)}$	CS_p is the chemical shift (mm) C_s is the chemical shift (3.5 ppm or 3.5×10^{-6}) γ is the gyromagnetic ratio (MHz/T) B_0 is the main magnetic field strength (T) FOV is the field of view in cm RBW is the receive bandwidth (Hz) Matrix(f) is the frequency matrix	This equation calculates the pixel shift in mm caused by the chemical shift between fat and water. To calculate the actual number of pixels that fat and water are shifted, remove the FOV function from this equation.

Appearance

Chemical shift artefact causes a signal void between areas of fat and water. Examples are around the kidneys, where the water-filled kidneys are surrounded by peri-renal fat, the orbits and vertebral bodies.

Remedy

- Scan with a low field-strength magnet.
- Remove either the fat or water signal by the use of STIR/chemical pre-saturation (see Chapters 16 and 40).
- Broaden the receive bandwidth – what is the trade-off? (See Chapter 34.)

Out-of-phase artefact is caused by the difference in precessional frequency between fat and water, which results in their magnetic moments being in phase with each other at certain times and out of phase at others (Figure 42.2). This is analogous to the hands on a clock, which have different frequencies as they travel around the clock face. There are certain points when both hands are at the same phase and other times when they are not. When the signals from both fat and water are out of phase, they cancel each other out so that signal loss results. If an image is produced when fat and water are out of phase, an artefact called **out-of-phase artefact** results. The time interval between fat and water being in phase is called the **periodicity**. This time depends on the frequency shift and therefore the field strength. At 1.5 T the periodicity is 4.2 ms. At lower field strengths the periodicity of fat and water is shorter and at higher field strengths it is longer.

Appearance

An out-of-phase image produces an asymmetric edging effect (Figure 42.3). This artefact mainly occurs along the phase axis and causes a dark ring around structures that contain both fat and water. It is most prevalent in gradient echo sequences, because gradient rephasing cannot compensate for the phase difference.

Remedy

- Use SE or FSE/ TSE pulse sequences (which use RF rephasing pulses).
- Use a TE that matches the periodicity of fat and water so that the echo is generated when fat and water are in phase.

The **Dixon technique** involves selecting a TE at half the periodicity so that fat and water are out of phase. In this way the signal from fat is reduced. This technique is mainly effective in areas where water and fat coexist in a voxel (see Chapter 40).

The key points of this chapter are summarized in Table 42.2.

Table 42.2 Key points.

Things to remember:
Fat and water precess at different frequencies. This is 3.5 ppm and is called chemical shift.
Chemical shift causes a displacement of fat and water signals in the frequency direction of the image. This is dependant on the field strength, the receive bandwidth and the FOV.
Chemical shift also causes the magnetic moments of fat and water to be only in phase at certain times, called the periodicity. If images are acquired when the magnetic moments of fat and water are out of phase, a signal void occurs.
Artefacts and their remedies are summarized in Appendix 2.

Access Scan Tip 4 and the MCQs relating to this chapter on the book's companion website at www.ataglanceseries.com/mri

Access Animation 7.1 relating to this chapter at www.westbrookmriinpractice.com/animations.asp

43 Phase mismapping

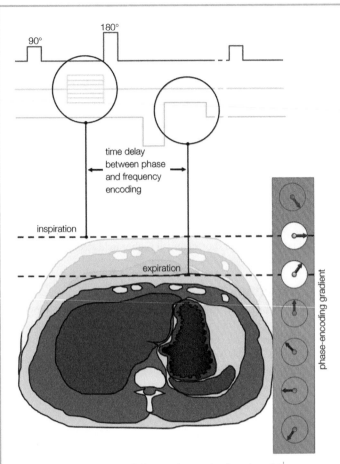

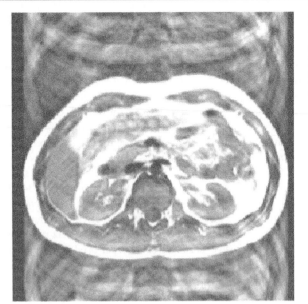

Figure 43.2 An axial image of the abdomen during breathing showing phase mismapping.

Figure 43.1 The cause of phase mismapping from breathing during the acquisition.

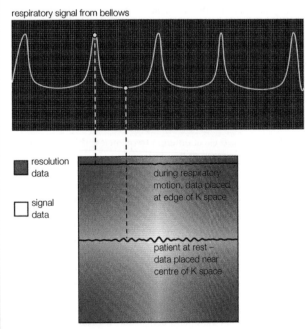

Figure 43.3 Respiratory compensation and K space.

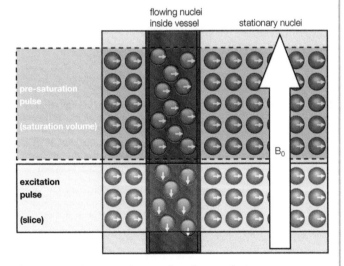

Figure 43.4 Pre-saturation to reduce flow artefact.

MRI at a Glance, Third Edition. Catherine Westbrook. © 2016 John Wiley & Sons, Ltd. Published 2016 by John Wiley & Sons, Ltd.

Companion website: www.ataglanceseries.com/mri

Motion artefact results from anatomy moving between the application of the phase-encoding gradient and the frequency-encoding gradient (intra-view) and motion between each application of the phase gradient (view to view). (See Scan Tip 12.) If anatomy moves during these periods it is assigned the wrong phase value and is mismapped onto the image. It causes an artefact called **ghosting** or **phase mismapping** and always occurs along the phase axis of the image.

The most common causes of phase mismapping are respiration, which moves the chest and abdominal wall along the phase-encoding gradient (Figure 43.1), and pulsatile movement of artery or vein walls or CSF. This type of motion is called periodic motion because it is regular in nature. Sudden movement of the patient during a scan is not the same type of motion. This is best avoided by taking time to position the patient carefully and immobilize them well.

Appearance

Blurring or ghosting across the image (Figure 43.2).

Remedy

There are many ways of reducing phase mismapping. These are described below.

Respiratory compensation

This specifically reduces phase mismapping from respiratory motion. In the simplest form, expandable air-filled **bellows** are placed around the patient's chest. The movement of air back and forth along the bellows during inspiration and expiration is converted to a waveform by a transducer. The system then orders the phase-encoding gradient so that the steep slopes occur when maximum movement of the chest wall occurs, and reserves the shallow gradient slopes (signal data) for minimum chest wall motion (Figure 49.3). In this way the motion does not appear to be periodic in terms of the data in K space and so phase mismapping artefact is reduced.

Other techniques to reduce phase mismapping from respiratory motion include breath-holding, where the patient holds their breath during the acquisition of data, and **respiratory triggering**, where data is only acquired when the chest wall is stationary. In this case the respiratory rate affects the scan time. A modification of this technique involves placing a small region of interest over the diaphragm on a sagittal or coronal image. As data is acquired during the sequence, the system tracks the motion of the diaphragm within the region of interest.

Cardiac and peripheral gating

Cardiac and peripheral gating uses gating leads or sensors to obtain an ECG trace of the patient's cardiac activity. The system acquires data from each slice at the same phase of the cardiac cycle, thereby reducing phase mismapping from cardiac and vessel pulsation. Cardiac gating is used when imaging the heart and great vessels. Peripheral gating is useful to reduce artefact from CSF flow.

Pre-saturation

Pre-saturation delivers a 90° RF pulse to a volume of tissue outside the FOV. This is called a **saturation band**. A flowing nucleus

within the volume receives this 90° pulse. When it enters the slice stack, it receives an excitation pulse and is saturated. If it is fully saturated to 180°, it has no transverse component of magnetization and produces a signal void (Figure 43.4). Therefore spins flowing into the slice have no signal to produce motion artefact. To be effective, pre-saturation pulses should be placed between the flow and the imaging stack, so that signal from flowing nuclei entering the FOV is nullified. Pre-saturation increases the rate of RF delivery to the patient; this increases the SAR.

Gradient moment nulling

Gradient moment rephasing or **nulling/flow compensation** for the altered phase values of the nuclei flowing along a gradient (see Chapter 53) uses additional gradients to correct the altered phases back to their original values. In this way, flowing nuclei do not gain, or lose, phase due to the presence of the main gradient and phase mismapping is reduced. Gradient moment rephasing gives flowing nuclei a bright signal, as they are in phase. Since gradient moment rephasing uses extra gradients, it increases the minimum TE.

Increasing NSA/NEX

Increasing NSA/NEX reduces phase mismapping by averaging noise data. Phase mismapping is a form of noise and therefore, by averaging this data, its appearance in the image is reduced (see Scan Tip 9). Propeller K space filling reduces motion artefact by signal averaging the centre of K space throughout the scan (see Chapter 38).

Swapping the phase and frequency direction so that artefact is removed from the area of interest does **not** eliminate mismapping; it only moves it away from the area of interest and, as such, is not considered a technique that eliminates this artefact (see Scan Tip 2).

Other remedies

• Bowel motion is reduced by giving the patient anti-spasmodic agents.
• Eye motion is reduced by asking the patient to fix their eyes on a particular point.

The key points of this chapter are summarized in Table 43.1.

Table 43.1 Key points.
Things to remember:
Phase mismapping, ghosting or motion artefact is caused by periodic motion, mainly as a result of spins moving between each phase encode.
It mainly originates from breathing and the pulsatile motion of vessels and CSF.
Respiratory compensation, gating, pre-saturation and gradient moment nulling are the main techniques used to reduce this artefact.
Artefacts and their remedies are summarized in Appendix 2.

 Access Scan Tips 2, 9 and 12 and the MCQs relating to this chapter on the book's companion website at **www.ataglanceseries.com/mri**

 Access Animation 6.3 relating to this chapter at **www .westbrookmriinpractice.com/animations.asp**

44 Aliasing

axial abdomen slice, spins exhibit phase curve after phase-encoding gradient application

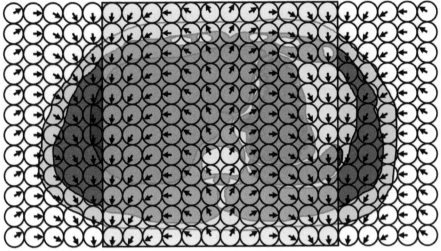

FOV

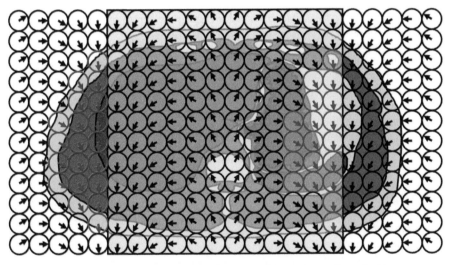

spins outside the field of view having same phase value as those inside

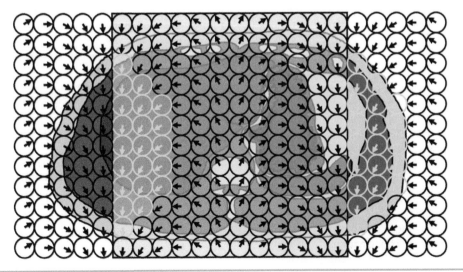

Figure 44.1 Aliasing or phase wrap.

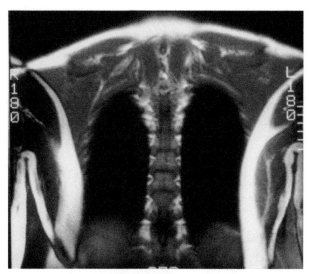

Figure 44.2 Coronal image of the chest showing aliasing.

liasing is caused by under-sampling of frequencies. If frequencies are not sampled often enough, the system cannot accurately represent those frequencies in the image. There is insufficient data in K space for the system to be able to accurately place signal that is produced from tissue outside of the FOV but within the coil. All tissue within the coil returns signal, but only frequencies within the FOV are used to produce the image. If there is insufficient data in K space, anatomy outside of the FOV is wrapped inside the FOV, ruining the image.

Frequency aliasing

In the frequency-encoding direction of the FOV, aliasing is avoided by ensuring that Nyquist is obeyed (see Chapter 34). If the digital sampling frequency is at least twice that of the highest frequency present in the FOV, then aliasing in the frequency-encoding direction of the image is avoided. In addition, low pass filters are used to remove unwanted frequencies.

Phase aliasing

Phase wrap/aliasing occurs when anatomy that is producing signal (as it is within the confines of the receiver coil) exists outside the FOV in the phase direction. Within the FOV, a finite number of phase values from 0° to 360° are mapped into the FOV in the phase direction. This can be represented as a 'phase curve' that is repeated on either side of the FOV in the phase direction if anatomy, which is producing signal, exists here. Due to the finite number of phase values, signal coming from outside the FOV has the same phase value as signal coming from inside, since they are both in the same position on the phase curve. There is therefore a duplication of phase values for anatomy inside and outside the FOV (Figure 44.1). It is caused by under-sampling of data when there are not enough data points in K space to accurately encode signal in the phase direction of the image.

Appearance

Anatomy outside the FOV in the phase direction is mapped onto the image. This is called **wrap around, fold over** or **aliasing**. Anatomy from one side of the image overlaps the other (Figure 44.2). Severe forms can ruin an image (see Scan Tip 2).

Remedy

Aliasing in the phase direction is reduced or eliminated in the following ways:

- Increasing the FOV to the boundaries of the coil.

- Placing spatial pre-saturation pulses over signal-producing anatomy.

Over-sampling in the phase direction is specifically called **anti-aliasing**. During data acquisition the FOV is increased in the phase direction, so that the phase curve extends over a larger FOV. There is now less likelihood of duplication of phase values of signal from anatomy outside the FOV, although, to achieve this, more phase-encoding steps must be performed. This increases the scan time. On some systems the NEX/NSA may be reduced to compensate for this. On these systems during image reconstruction the extra FOV is discarded (only the middle portion corresponding to the FOV selected is displayed). There is usually no penalty in scan time, signal or spatial resolution when using anti-aliasing on these systems, although motion artefact may be increased due to less signal averaging (see Chapter 43).

On other systems the phase FOV is extended to cover anatomy in the phase-encoding direction. This causes the scan time to increase proportionally. The NSA or NEX may be reduced to compensate for this. Although decreasing the NSA or NEX reduces the SNR, over-sampling of data by using anti-aliasing software compensates for this (see Scan Tip 9).

Did you know?

The Nyquist theorem states that in order to represent a frequency accurately, it must be sampled at least twice as frequently. In the echo there are hundreds of different frequencies. The range or bandwidth of frequencies received during the sampling time is called the receive bandwidth, and when Nyquist is obeyed the digital sampling frequency is twice as high as the highest frequency in the bandwidth. The receive bandwidth is commonly represented as a +/− frequency relative to the centre frequency of the echo; for example, +/− 16 KHz, meaning that the receive bandwidth is 32 KHz in total. If Nyquist is obeyed, the digital sampling frequency is 2 × 16 KHz (the highest frequency in the bandwidth), which is 32 KHz. Thus the receive bandwidth has the same numerical value as the digital sampling rate. On the MR system the digital sampling frequency is therefore controlled by altering the receive bandwidth (see Chapter 34).

Not sampling often enough causes aliasing. An example is watching a film of a wheel turning, such as a car advert or a wagon wheel in an old-fashioned Western film. The wheel sometimes looks stationary or like it is moving backwards. That is because the frame rate of the camera is not fast enough for certain velocities of the rotating wheel.

The key points of this chapter are summarized in Table 44.1.

Table 44.1 Key points.

Things to remember:
Aliasing is caused by under-sampling of frequencies.
If frequencies are not sampled often enough, the system cannot accurately represent those frequencies in the image.
In the frequency-encoding direction of the image, this is avoided by ensuring that the digital sampling frequency is at least twice that of the highest frequency present and additional low-pass filters are used.
In the phase-encoding direction of the image, aliasing is remedied by using anti-aliasing software.
Artefacts and their remedies are summarized in Appendix 2.

Access Scan Tips 2 and 9 and the MCQs relating to this chapter on the book's companion website at www.ataglanceseries.com/mri

45 Other artefacts

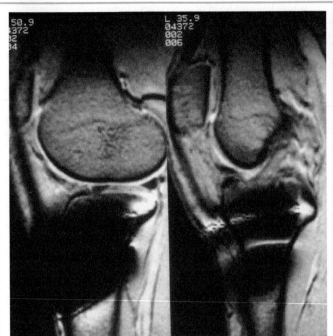

Figure 45.1 Sagittal GE imaging of the knee with metal screws in place. Magnetic susceptibility artefact is clearly seen.

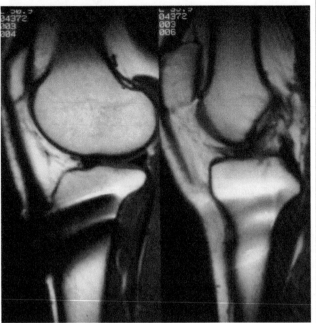

Figure 45.2 Same patient as in Figure 45.1 using a spin echo sequence. The artefact is reduced because RF rephasing corrects for differences in susceptibility between structures.

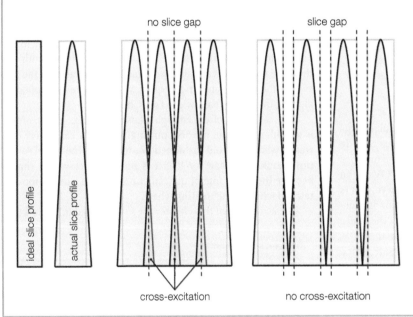

ideal slice profile

actual slice profile

no slice gap

slice gap

cross-excitation

no cross-excitation

Figure 45.3 Cross-talk.

MRI at a Glance, Third Edition. Catherine Westbrook. © 2016 John Wiley & Sons, Ltd. Published 2016 by John Wiley & Sons, Ltd.
Companion website: www.ataglanceseries.com/mri

Magnetic susceptibility

Magnetic susceptibility artefact occurs because all tissues magnetize to a different degree depending on their magnetic characteristics (see Chapter 1). This produces a difference in their individual precessional frequencies and phase. The phase discrepancy causes dephasing at the boundaries of structures with very different magnetic susceptibility, and signal loss results.

Appearance

This artefact appears as areas of signal void and high signal intensity, often accompanied by distortion. It is commonly seen on gradient echo sequences when the patient has a metal prosthesis in situ, because gradient rephasing cannot compensate for these magnetic field distortions (Figure 45.1). Magnetic susceptibility also occurs naturally, such as at the interface of the petrous bone and the brain. Magnetic susceptibility can be used advantageously when investigating haemorrhage or blood products, as the presence of this artefact suggests that bleeding has recently occurred.

Remedy

Employ SE or TSE pulse sequences that use RF rephasing pulses (Figure 45.2). Remove all metal items from the patient before the examination.

Cross-talk

Cross-talk is caused by the fact that RF pulses and their Fourier transforms are not exactly square. They are usually Gaussian in shape and therefore have side lobes so that they are wider than the slice (Figure 45.3; note that cross-talk is referred to as cross-exception in this diagram). Therefore when two slices are adjacent to each other, there is an overlap in their RF pulses that causes the effective TR of each slice to decrease. This occurs because spins in the overlap are saturated by RF excitation pulses in adjacent slices.

Appearance

Adjacent slices have different image contrasts. T1 weighting is increased and SNR decreased due to saturation.

Remedy

Gaps are introduced between slices so that there is no overlap of RF excitation pulses and their Fourier transforms. This, however, means that some anatomy is missed, so it is important to select this parameter carefully. A slice gap of 30% of the slice thickness is optimal rather than a slice gap of 10%, unless using squared-off RF pulses.

The slices may be interleaved or concatenated. This means that the system performs two acquisitions: one acquiring odd slices and another even slices. This doubles the scan time, although as only half the number of slices are being acquired per acquisition, it is usually possible to reduce the TR when interleaving. This technique reduces cross-talk because there is a whole slice thickness between each slice. Most systems square off the RF pulses so that their profiles more accurately fit the rectangular profile of the slice. This allows a slice gap of 10% without cross-talk. However, this results in a loss of signal, as a proportion of the RF pulse is lost during the squaring-off process.

Truncation artefact

Truncation artefact is caused by under-sampling because too few K space lines are filled. This occurs when the phase matrix is very low or when a K space filling technique that only partly fills K space is used, such as partial averaging (see Chapter 38). When there is insufficient data in K space, the system cannot accurately represent the borders of very high and very low signal and a banding artefact is produced.

Appearance

A banding artefact is seen at the boundaries of very high and very low signal, such as a very high signal from fat in the scalp adjacent to the very low signal from cortical bone on the skull in T1 or PD weighted images. It occurs in the phase direction and produces a low signal intensity band running through a high signal intensity area.

Remedy

Increase the number of phase-encoding steps and avoid partial K space filling techniques.

Zipper artefact

Zipper artefact is caused by extraneous RF of entering the scan room and interfering with the relatively weak signal from the patient. It is usually caused by a leak in the RF shielding of the scan room that permits RF of a particular frequency to enter the room.

Appearance

Zipper artefact appears as a line across the image in the frequency-encoding axis. Its position depends on the frequency of the interference.

Remedy

Locate the source of the leak and repair it.

The key points of this chapter are summarized in Table 45.1.

Table 45.1 Key points.
Things to remember:
Magnetic susceptibility is caused by different tissues being magnetized differently. It is reduced by using spin echo sequences. Sometimes it is a good artefact in that it increases the conspicuity of haemorrhage when using gradient echo sequences.
Truncation is caused by under-sampling of phase data. It is remedied by filling more of K space.
Cross-talk is caused by the non-rectangular profile of RF pulses and their Fourier transforms. One of the ways to remedy this is to introduce a gap or skip between slices.
Artefacts and their remedies are summarized in Appendix 2.

Access the MCQs relating to this chapter on the book's companion website at **www.ataglanceseries.com/mri**

46 Flow phenomena

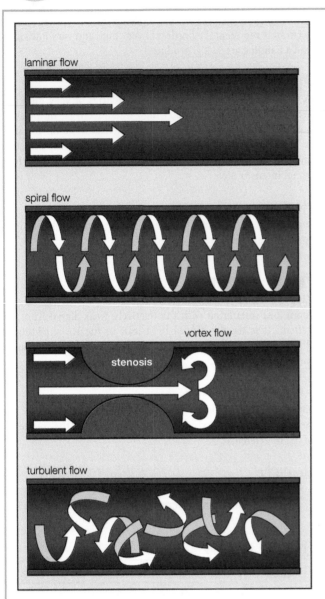

laminar flow

spiral flow

vortex flow

stenosis

turbulent flow

Figure 46.1 The different types of flow.

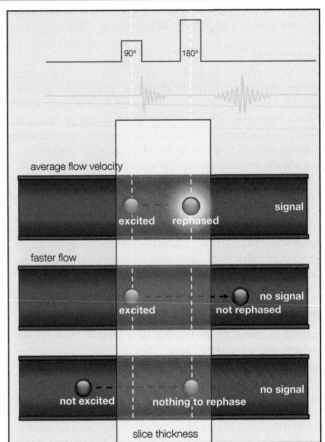

average flow velocity

excited   rephased   signal

faster flow

excited   not rephased   no signal

not excited   nothing to rephase   no signal

slice thickness

Figure 46.2 Time-of-flight flow phenomenon.

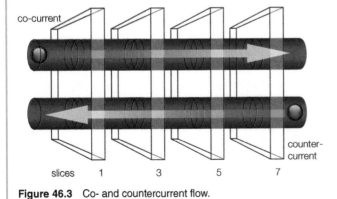

co-current

slices   1   3   5   7

counter-current

Figure 46.3 Co- and countercurrent flow.

stationary nucleus

gradient on

flowing nucleus gains phase

Figure 46.4 Intra-voxel dephasing.

MRI at a Glance, Third Edition. Catherine Westbrook. © 2016 John Wiley & Sons, Ltd. Published 2016 by John Wiley & Sons, Ltd.

Companion website: www.ataglanceseries.com/mri

*L*aminar flow is flow that is at different but consistent velocities across a vessel. The flow at the centre of the lumen of the vessel is faster than at the vessel wall, where resistance slows down the flow. However, the velocity difference across the vessel is constant.

Turbulent flow is flow at different velocities that fluctuates randomly. The velocity difference across the vessel changes erratically.

Vortex flow is flow that is initially laminar, but then passes through a stricture or stenosis in the vessel. Flow in the centre of the lumen has a high velocity, but near the walls the flow spirals (Figure 46.1). (See Table 46.1.)

Table 46.1 Equations of flow phenomena.

Equations (if you like them)		
$Re = dvm/vis$	Re is the Reynolds number d is density (g/cm³) v is velocity of flow (cm/s) m is the diameter of the vessel (cm) vis is the viscosity of blood (g/cm-s)	If Re is less than 2100 then flow is laminar. If Re is more than 2100 then flow is turbulent.
$SI \alpha 1-v(1/2TE)/S_t$	SI is the signal intensity v is velocity of flow (cm/s) TE is the echo time (ms) S_t is the slice thickness (cm)	This equation shows how the time-of-flight effect depends on TE, slice thickness and velocity of flow.
$v = S_t/TR$	v is the velocity of flow (cm/s) St is the slice thickness (cm) TR is the repetition time (ms)	This equation calculates the velocity of flow required to replace all the saturated spins in a slice with fresh unsaturated spins.

Time-of-flight phenomenon

In order to produce a signal, a nucleus must receive an excitation pulse and a rephasing pulse. Stationary nuclei always receive both excitation and rephasing pulses. Flowing nuclei present in the slice for the excitation may have exited the slice before rephasing. This is called **time-of-flight phenomenon**. If a nucleus receives the excitation pulse only and is not rephased, it does not produce a signal. If a nucleus is rephased but has not previously been excited, it does not produce a signal (Figure 46.2). Time-of-flight effects depend on:
- velocity of flow;
- TE;
- slice thickness.

Flow-related enhancement increases as:
- velocity of flow decreases;
- TE decreases;
- slice thickness increases.

High-velocity signal loss increases as:
- velocity of flow increases;
- TE increases;
- slice thickness decreases.

Entry slice phenomenon

Entry slice phenomenon (also known as the in-flow effect) is related to the excitation history of the nuclei. Nuclei that receive repeated RF pulses during the acquisition are saturated. Nuclei that have not received these repeated RF pulses are 'fresh', as their magnetic moments have not been saturated by successive RF pulses. The signal that they produce is different to that of the saturated nuclei.

Stationary nuclei within a slice become saturated after repeated RF pulses. Nuclei flowing perpendicular to the slice enter the slice fresh, as they were not present during repeated excitations. They therefore produce a different signal to the stationary nuclei. This is called entry slice phenomenon, as it is most prominent in the first slice of a 'stack' of slices. The slices in the middle of the stack exhibit less entry slice phenomenon, as flowing nuclei have received more excitation pulses by the time they reach these slices. The magnitude of entry slice phenomenon therefore depends on:
- TR;
- slice thickness;
- velocity of flow;
- direction of flow.

Direction of flow

Co-current flow: Flow that is in the *same* direction as slice selection is called *co-current*. The flowing nuclei are more likely to receive repeated RF excitations as they move from one slice to the next. They therefore become saturated relatively quickly, and so entry slice phenomenon decreases rapidly.

Countercurrent flow: Flow that is in the *opposite* direction to slice selection is called *countercurrent* flow. Flowing nuclei stay fresh, as when they enter a slice they are less likely to have received previous excitation pulses (Figure 46.3). Entry slice phenomenon does not therefore decrease rapidly and may still be present deep within the slice stack.

Intra-voxel dephasing

Nuclei flowing along a gradient rapidly accelerate or decelerate depending on the direction of flow. Flowing nuclei either gain phase or lose phase or lose phase (See Figure 46.4.) If a flowing nucleus is adjacent to a stationary nucleus in a voxel, there is a phase difference between the two nuclei. This is because the flowing nucleus has either lost or gained phase relative to the stationary nucleus due to its motion along the gradient. Nuclei within the same voxel are out of phase with each other, which results in a reduction of total signal amplitude from the voxel. This is called **intra-voxel dephasing**.

The key points of this chapter are summarized in Table 46.2.

Table 46.2 Key points.

Things to remember:
Only laminar flow can be compensated for, as it is the only type of flow that is regular.
Time-of-flight flow phenomenon is caused by nuclei not being excited and rephased. It therefore depends on the velocity of low, the slice thickness and the TE.
Entry slice phenomenon is caused by saturation of flowing spins due to repeated excitation. It depends mainly on the velocity of flow, the TR and the direction of flow relative to slice excitation.
Intra-voxel dephasing occurs when spins move along a gradient and therefore have a different phase than stationary spins in the same voxel. It depends on the TE and TR.
See Appendix 2 for methods used to compensate for flow phenomena.

Access Animations 6.1, 6.2 and 6.3 relating to this chapter at www.westbrookmriinpractice.com/animations.asp

Time-of-flight MR angiography

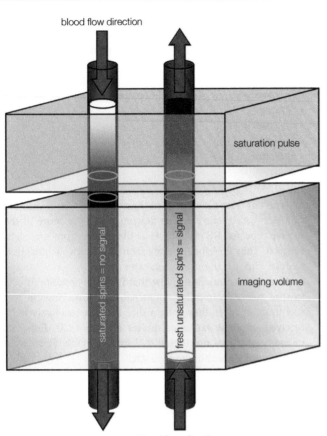

Figure 47.1 Presaturation volume relative to the imaging stack.

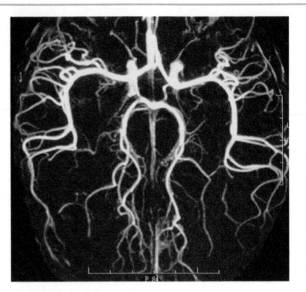

Figure 47.3 3D TOF MRA of a 4-year-old child showing normal appearances.

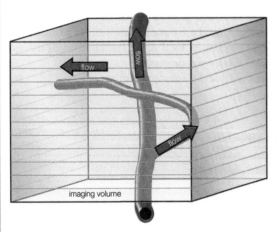

Figure 47.2 Flow and the imaging volume.

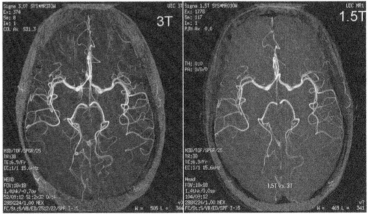

Figure 47.4 Axial 3D TOF-MRA of the brain acquired at 3 T (left) and 1.5 T (right). Note the enhanced SNR and CNR of the 3 T image.

Mechanism

Time-of-flight MRA or **TOF MRA** produces vascular contrast by manipulating longitudinal magnetization of stationary spins. It uses a gradient echo pulse sequence in combination with gradient moment rephasing to enhance signal in flowing vessels. The TR is kept well below the T1 time of the stationary tissues so that T1 recovery is prevented. This saturates the stationary spins, while the inflow effect from fully magnetized flowing fresh spins produces high vascular signal (see Chapter 46). However, if the TR is too short, the flowing spins may be suppressed along with the stationary spins, and that has the effect of reducing vascular contrast. To evaluate signals from arterial flow, saturation pulses are applied in the direction of venous flow. For example, to evaluate the carotid arteries in the neck, apply saturation pulses superior to the imaging volume to saturate the signal from inflowing venous blood (see Chapter 43 and Figure 47.1). TOF MRA is only sensitive to flow that comes into the FOV. Any flow that traverses the FOV can be saturated along with the stationary tissue (Figure 47.2).

2D vs 3D time-of-flight MRA

TOF MRA is acquired in either 2D (slice by slice) or 3D (volume) acquisition modes. In general, 3D volume imaging offers high SNR and thin contiguous slices for good resolution. However, as TOF MRA is sensitive to flow coming into the FOV or the imaging volume, spins in vessels with slow flow can be saturated in volume imaging. For this reason, 3D TOF should be used in areas of high-velocity flow (intracranial applications) and 2D TOF in areas of slower-velocity flow (carotids, peripheral vascular and the venous systems). In 3D techniques, there is a higher risk of saturating signals from spins within the volume.

Clinical applications

The carotid bifurcation, the peripheral circulation and cortical venous mapping can be imaged with 2D TOF MRA (Figures 47.3 and 47.4).

Typical values

- TR: 45 ms
- TE: minimum allowable
- Flip angle: approx. 60°
- The TR and flip angle saturate stationary nuclei, but moving spins coming into the slice remain fresh, so image contrast is maximized.
- The short TE reduces phase mismapping.
- Gradient moment rephasing, in conjunction with saturation pulses to suppress signals from areas of undesired flow, is used to enhance vascular contrast.

General advantages of TOF MRA

- Sensitive to T1 effects (short T1 tissues are bright; contrast may be given for additional enhancement).
- Reasonable imaging times (approximately 5 minutes depending on parameters).
- Sensitive to slow flow.
- Reduced sensitivity to intra-voxel dephasing.

General disadvantages of TOF MRA

- Sensitive to T1 effects (short T1 tissues are bright so that haemorrhagic lesions may mimic vessels).
- Saturation of in-plane flow (any flow within the FOV or volume of tissue can be saturated along with background tissue).
- Enhancement is limited to either flow entering the FOV or very high-velocity flow (Tables 47.1 and 47.2).

Table 47.1 Comparison of advantages and disadvantages of 2D and 3D time-of-flight MRA.

Advantages of 2D TOF MRA	Disadvantages of 2D TOF MRA
Large area of coverage	Lower resolution
Sensitive to slow flow	Saturation of in-plane flow
Sensitive to T1 effects	Venetian blind artefact

Advantages of 3D TOF MRA	Disadvantages of 3D TOF MRA
High resolution for small vessels	Saturation of in-plane flow
Sensitive to T1 effects	Small area of coverage

Table 47.2 Overcoming disadvantages of time-of-flight MRA.

Susceptibility artefacts	Use short TEs and small voxel volumes
Poor background suppression	Use a TE that acquires data when fat and water are out of phase Implement magnetization transfer techniques
Venetian blind artefacts	Use breath-hold techniques
Limited coverage (3D)	Acquire images in another plane Use MOTSA (multiple overlapping thin-section angiography)
Suppression of in-plane signal	Use ramped RF pulses Administer contrast media
Pulsation artefacts	Time acquisition to the cardiac cycle

The key points of this chapter are summarized in Table 47.3.

Table 47.3 Key points.

Things to remember:
Time-of-flight angiography is *not* the same as time-of-flight flow phenomenon.
TOF-MRA is a technique that produces images where unsaturated spins coming into the slice produce a higher signal intensity than the stationary spins within the slice.
Saturation pulses are also used to null signal from unwanted flow (venous).
3D TOF-MRA is useful in high-velocity flow regions. 2D TOF-MRA is useful in slower flow regions.

48 Phase contrast MR angiography

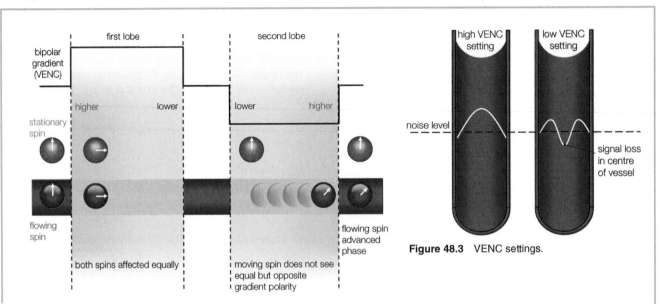

Figure 48.1 Bipolar gradients in phase contrast MRA.

first lobe

second lobe

bipolar gradient (VENC)

higher   lower   lower   higher

stationary spin

flowing spin

both spins affected equally

moving spin does not see equal but opposite gradient polarity

flowing spin advanced phase

high VENC setting   low VENC setting

noise level

signal loss in centre of vessel

Figure 48.3   VENC settings.

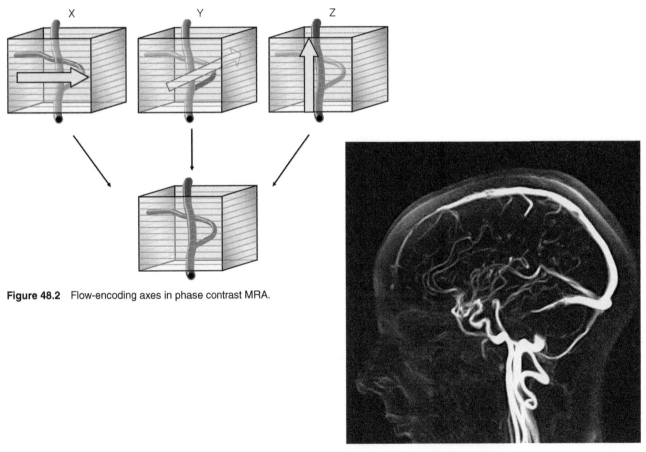

Figure 48.2   Flow-encoding axes in phase contrast MRA.

Figure 48.4   PC venogram of the brain.

Mechanism

Phase contrast MRA utilizes velocity changes, and hence phase shifts in moving spins, to provide image contrast in flowing vessels. Phase shifts are generated in the pulse sequence by phase encoding the velocity of flow with the use of a bipolar (two lobes – one negative, one positive) gradient. Phase shift is introduced selectively for moving spins with the use of gradients. This technique is known as phase contrast magnetic resonance angiography or **PC MRA**. PC MRA is sensitive to flow within, as well as that coming into, the FOV.

Immediately after the RF excitation pulse, spins are in phase. A gradient is applied to both stationary and flowing spins. Although phase shifts occur in both stationary and flowing spins, these shifts occur at different rates. During initial application of the first bipolar gradient, there is a shift of phases of stationary spins and flowing spins.

After the second part of the application of the first bipolar gradient, the stationary spins return to their initial phase, but those of moving spins acquire some phase (Figure 48.1). The bipolar gradient is then applied with opposite polarity so that the same variants occur, but in the opposite direction.

PC MRA then subtracts the two acquisitions so that the signals from stationary spins are subtracted out, leaving only the signals from flowing spins. The combination of PC MRA acquisitions results in what are known as magnitude and phase images. The unsubtracted combinations of flow-sensitized image data are known as *magnitude* images. The subtracted combinations are called *phase* images.

The bipolar gradients induce phase shifts along their axes. By applying bipolar gradients in all three axes, the sequence is sensitized to flow in all three directions, X, Y and Z. These are known as **flow-encoding axes** (Figure 48.2). The sequence is also sensitized to flow velocity using a **velocity-encoding technique** or **VENC**, which compensates for projected flow velocity within vessels by controlling the amplitude or strength of the bipolar gradient. If the VENC selected is lower than the velocity within the vessel, aliasing can occur. This results in low signal intensity in the centre of the vessel, but better delineation of the vessel wall itself. With high VENC settings, intraluminal signal is improved, but vessel wall delineation is compromised (Figure 48.3).

2D vs 3D phase contrast MRA

2D techniques provide acceptable imaging times and flow direction information. 2D acquisitions, however, cannot be reformatted and viewed in other imaging planes. 3D offers SNR and spatial resolution superior to 2D imaging strategies, and the ability to reformat in a number of imaging planes retrospectively. The trade-off, however, is that in 3D PC MRA, imaging time increases with the TR, NSA, the number of phase-encoding steps, the number of slices and the number of flow-encoding axes selected. For this reason, scan times are sometimes long (Table 48.1).

Table 48.1 Advantages and disadvantages of phase contrast MRA.

Advantages	Disadvantages
Sensitivity to a variety of vascular velocities	Long imaging times with 3D
Sensitivity to flow within the FOV	More sensitive to turbulence
Reduced intra-voxel dephasing	
Increased background suppression	
Magnitude and phase images	

Clinical uses

Phase contrast MRA can be used effectively in the evaluation of arteriovenous malformations, aneurysms, venous occlusions, congenital abnormalities and traumatic intracranial vascular injuries (Figure 48.4).

Typical values

3D volume acquisitions
- Slices: 28 slices volume, 1 mm slice thickness
- Flip angle: 20° (60-slice volume flip angle reduced to 15°)
- TR: ≤25 ms
- VENC: 40–60 cm/s
- Flow encoding: in all directions

2D techniques acquisitions
Cranial
- TR: 18–20 ms
- Flip angle: 20°
- Slices: thickness 20–60 mm
- VENC: 20–30 cm/s for venous flow
- 40–60 cm/s for higher velocity with some aliasing
- 60–80 cm/s to determine velocity and flow direction

Carotid
- Flip angle: 20–30°
- TR: 20 ms
- VENC: 40–60 cm/s for better morphology with aliasing
- 60–80 cm/s for quantitative velocity and directional information

The key points of this chapter are summarized in Table 48.2.

Table 48.2 Key points.

Things to remember:

PC-MRA uses gradients to sensitize the sequence to flow. Flowing spins have a higher signal than stationary spins.

The amplitude of the sensitizing gradients is controlled by the VENC. If the VENC is too low aliasing occurs. If the VENC is high then vessel wall delineation may be compromised.

3D PC-MRA produces images with a better SNR and spatial resolution than 2D, but the scan times are long.

49 Contrast-enhanced MR angiography

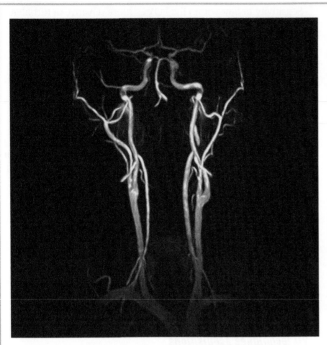

Figure 49.1 Coronal CE MRA of the carotid and vertebral arteries.

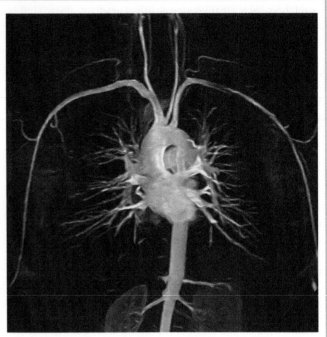

Figure 49.2 Coronal CE MRA of the chest.

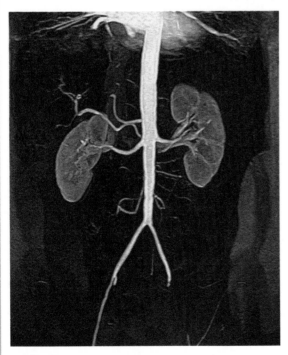

Figure 49.3 Coronal CE MRA of the abdominal vessels.

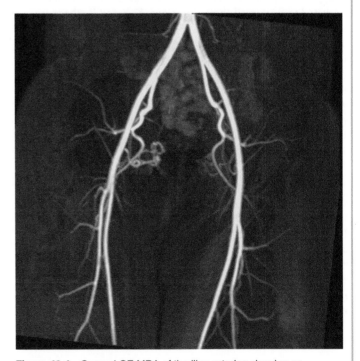

Figure 49.4 Coronal CE MRA of the iliac arteries showing an arteriovenous malformation.

Mechanism

Gadolinium is a T1 shortening agent that enhances blood if given in sufficient quantities into the bloodstream. If used in conjunction with a T1 weighted sequence, blood appears bright and is well seen in contrast to surrounding non-enhancing tissues (see Chapter 50; Table 49.1; Figures 49.1, 49.2, 49.3 and 49.4). A conventional or fast incoherent gradient echo sequence should be used to keep scan times short (see Chapters 21 and 24).

Table 49.1 Advantages and disadvantages of contrast-enhanced MRA.

Advantages	Disadvantages
Easier to visualize vessels – fewer false positives	Timing is sometimes difficult
No extra sequences needed	Invasive – risk of reaction
With practice, examination complete in 15–30 mins	Extra equipment such as power injectors and moving tables may be required

Administration

Administration is intravenous, usually via the ante-cubital fossa by hand or mechanical injection. Doses must be sufficiently high to give adequate visualization of vessels; 40–60 ml (about 0.3 mmol/kg) of gadolinium is required.

Image timing

Timing is essential for contrast-enhanced MRA (CE-MRA). To obtain an arterial-phase image in which arteries are bright and veins are dark, it is essential that the central K space data (i.e. the low spatial frequency data) is acquired while gadolinium concentration in the arteries is high but relatively lower in the veins (see Chapter 38).

The time it takes contrast to travel from the ante-cubital fossa to the area of interest depends on:
- distance of the area from the injection site;
- type of vessel (e.g. artery or vein);
- velocity of flow;
- speed of injection;
- length of the acquisition.

For long acquisitions, lasting more than 100 s, use sequential ordering of K space, so that the centre of K space is collected first (**centric K space filling**; see Chapter 38). Sequential ordering results in fewer artefacts. Begin injecting the gadolinium just after initiating imaging. Finish the injection just after the midpoint of the acquisition, being careful to maintain the maximum injection rate for the approximately 10–30 s prior to the middle of the acquisition. This will ensure a maximum arterial gadolinium during the middle of the acquisition when central K space data is collected.

For short acquisitions, less than 45 s, contrast agent bolus timing is more critical and challenging. There are several approaches to determining the optimal bolus timing for these fast scans. For a typical breath-hold scan duration of 35–45 s in a reasonably healthy patient with an intravenous site in the ante-cubital vein, a delay of approximately 10–12 s is appropriate. Therefore, begin the injection, and then 10 s later start imaging while the patient suspends breathing.

More reliable and precise techniques are also available. These include the following:
- Using a test bolus to precisely measure the contrast travel time.
- Using an automatic pulse sequence that monitors signal in the aorta and then initiates imaging after contrast is detected arriving in the aorta. This is called bolus tracking, where a tracker pulse is positioned to measure signal within the lumen of the aorta or large vessel proximal to the imaging volume. The scan is initialized when increased signal from the contrast agent is detected. Another automated option called 'fluoro' triggering uses a navigator-type acquisition to initiate the scan providing good temporal resolution.
- Imaging so rapidly that bolus timing is unimportant.

CE-MRA images can be post-processed with Maximum Intensity Projection (MIP) or Shaded Surface Display (SSD).

MIP assigns a numerical value to each pixel in terms of its greyscale and then projects the maximum intensity for each row or column within each slice in a 2D plane. These images permit visualization of flow from different angles, but provide a rather flat perspective. It is sometimes difficult to tell which vessels lie at the front and which lie behind.

SSD improves the perception of the data by using Phong's formula. It segments the data using edge detection so that edges look like surfaces illuminated by a directional light source. The benefit of this is that vessels closer to the observer appear to lie in front of structures that lie behind.

Both MIP and SSD can be used in TOF-MRA (see Chapter 47). If the background is not suppressed enough using these techniques, then subtraction techniques can be used. These take an image without contrast and subtract it from the contrast-enhanced image.

The key points of this chapter are summarized in Table 49.2.

Table 49.2 Key points.

Things to remember:
CE-MRA uses the T1 shortening properties of gadolinium to label flow spins within a vessel.
Flow appears bright and non-flow is suppressed by using MIP, SSD or subtraction techniques.
Timing is very important to ensure that the centre of K space is filled when gadolinium enters the imaging volume.

50 Contrast agents

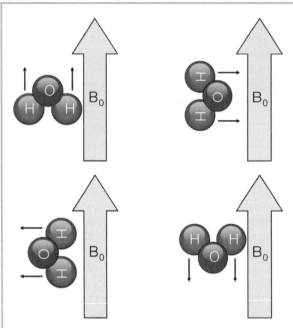

Figure 50.1 Tumbling of water molecules.

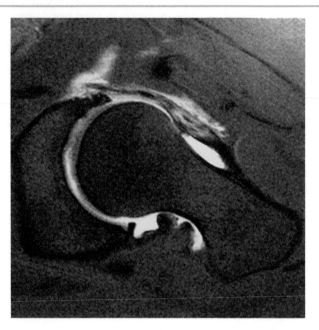

Figure 50.2 Axial arthrogram of the hip using gadolinium.

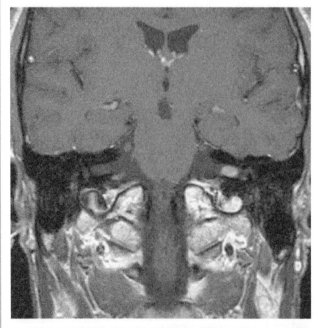

Figure 50.3 Coronal T1 weighted image of a small left acoustic neuroma after administration of gadolinium.

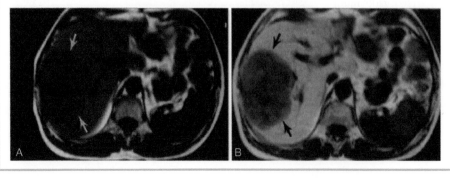

Figure 50.4 Axial T1 weighted image of the liver without (left) and with (right) manganese contrast. The enhanced image shows enhancement of normal liver so that the liver pathology is darker.

MRI at a Glance, Third Edition. Catherine Westbrook. © 2016 John Wiley & Sons, Ltd. Published 2016 by John Wiley & Sons, Ltd.
Companion website: www.ataglanceseries.com/mri

I n order to increase contrast between pathology and normal tissue, enhancement agents may be introduced that selectively affect the T1 and T2 relaxation times in tissues (see Chapter 40). Both T1 recovery and T2 decay are influenced by the magnetic field experienced locally within the nucleus. The local magnetic field responsible for these processes is caused by:

- the main magnetic field;
- fluctuations as a result of the magnetic moments of nuclear spins in neighbouring molecules.

These molecules rotate or tumble, and the rate of rotation of the molecules is a characteristic property of the solution. It is dependent on:

- magnetic field strength;
- viscosity of the solution;
- temperature of the solution.

Molecules that tumble with a frequency at or near the Larmor frequency have more efficient T1 recovery times than other molecules (Figure 50.1).

The phenomenon by which excited protons are affected by nearby excited protons and electrons is called **dipole-dipole** interaction. If a tumbling molecule with a large magnetic moment such as gadolinium is placed in the presence of water protons, local magnetic field fluctuations occur near the Larmor frequency. T1 relaxation times of nearby protons are therefore reduced and so they appear bright on a T1 weighted image. This effect on a substance whereby relaxation rates are altered is known as **relaxivity**.

Gadolinium

Gadolinium (Gd) is a **paramagnetic** agent. It is a trivalent lanthanide element that has seven unpaired electrons and an ability to allow rapid exchange of bulk water to minimize the space between itself and water within the body. It has a large magnetic moment and, when it is placed in the presence of tumbling water protons, fluctuations in the local magnetic field are created near the Larmor frequency. The T1 relaxation times of nearby water protons are therefore reduced, resulting in an increased signal intensity on T1 weighted images. For this reason, gadolinium is known as a **T1 enhancement agent**.

Chelation

Gadolinium is a rare earth metal that cannot be excreted by the body and would cause long-term side effects as it binds to membranes. By binding the gadolinium ion to a chelate such as diethylene triaminepentaacetic acid (DTPA, a ligand), the chelate compound Gd-DTPA is formed, which can be safely excreted.

Administration

The effective dosage of Gd-DTPA is 0.1 millimoles per kilogram of body weight (mmol/kg) – approximately 0.2 ml/kg or 0.1 ml/lb – with a maximum dose of 20 ml.

Clinical applications

Gadolinium has proven invaluable in imaging the central nervous system because of its ability to pass through breakdowns in the blood–brain barrier (BBB). Clinical indications for gadolinium include:

- tumours (Figure 50.3);
- infection;
- arthrography (Figure 50.2);
- post-operation lumbar disc;
- breast disease;
- vessel patency and morphology (see Chapter 49).

Iron oxide

Iron oxides shorten relaxation times of nearby hydrogen atoms and therefore reduce the signal intensity in normal tissues. This results in a signal loss on proton density weighted or heavily T2 weighted images. Super-paramagnetic iron oxides are known as **T2 enhancement agents**. Iron oxide is taken up by the reticulo-endothelial system and excreted by the liver, so that normal liver is dark and liver lesions are bright on T2 weighted images.

Administration

The recommended dose of iron oxide is 0.56 mg of iron per kg of body weight. This should be diluted in 100 ml of 50% dextrose and given intravenously over 30 mins. The diluted drug is administered through a 5-micron filter at a rate of 2–4 mmol/min. This agent should be used within 8 hours following dilution.

Clinical applications

Iron oxide is mainly used in liver and biliary imaging (Figure 50.4).

Other contrast agents

Gastrointestinal contrast agents are sometimes used for bowel enhancement. These include barium, ferromagnetic agents and fatty substances. However, due to constant peristalsis, these agents enhance bowel motion artefacts more often than enhancing pathological lesions. The use of anti-spasmodic agents helps to retard peristalsis to decrease these artefacts. Other agents include helium, which is inhaled and assists in the evaluation of lung perfusion.

The key points of this chapter are summarized in Table 50.1.

Table 50.1 Key points.

Things to remember:
The purpose of contrast agents is to ensure that pathology has a different contrast to surrounding normal anatomy.
Contrast agents are either T1 or T2 enhancement agents.
The effect of altering the relaxivity rates of tissues by administering a contrast agent is called relaxivity.

51 Magnets

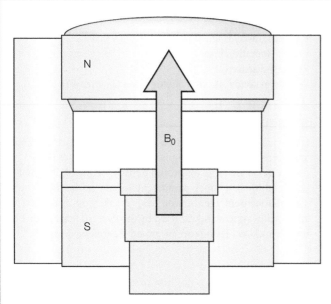

Figure 51.1 A permanent magnet.

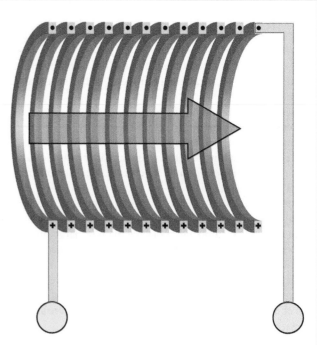

Figure 51.2 A simple electromagnet.

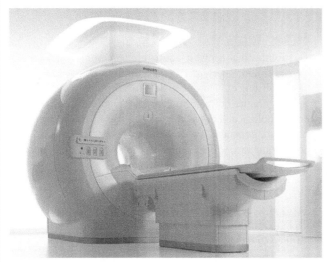

Figure 51.3 A superconducting system.

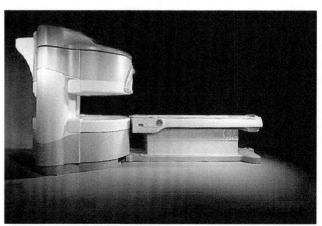

Figure 51.4 A high field open system.

Permanent magnets

Permanent magnets consist of ferromagnetic substances that have magnetic susceptibility greater than 1. They are easily magnetized and retain this magnetization (Figure 51.1). Examples of substances used are iron, cobalt and nickel. The most common material used is an alloy of aluminium, nickel and cobalt, known as **alnico**.

Advantages

Open design: children, obese and claustrophobic patients scanned with ease. Interventional and dynamic procedures are possible. They require no power supply, and operating costs are therefore low. The magnetic field created by a permanent magnet has lines of flux running vertically, keeping the magnetic field virtually confined within the boundaries of the scan room.

Disadvantages

Excessive weight, only low fixed field strengths (0.2–0.3 T) can be achieved. Longer scan times due to lower field strengths.

Electromagnets

Electromagnets utilize the laws of electromagnetic induction by passing an electrical current through a series of wires to produce a magnetic field (see Chapter 1). This physical phenomenon is utilized to produce RF coils and the static magnetic field.

Resistive magnets

The magnetic field strength in a resistive magnet is dependent on the current that passes through its coils of wire. The direction of the main magnetic field in a resistive magnet follows the right-hand thumb rule and produces lines of flux running horizontally from the head to the foot of the magnet (see Chapter 1 and Figure 51.2).

Advantages

They are lighter in weight than permanent magnets and capital costs are low.

Disadvantages

The operational costs of the resistive magnet are quite high due to the large quantities of power required to maintain the magnetic field. The maximum field strength in a system of this type is less than 0.3 T due to its excessive power requirements. Therefore scan times are longer. The resistive system is relatively safe, as the field can be turned off instantaneously. However, this type of magnet does create significant stray fringe magnetic fields.

Superconducting electromagnets

The resistance of the coils of wire is dependent on the material of which the loops of wire are made, the length of the wire in the loop, the cross-sectional area of the wire and temperature. The latter can be controlled so that resistance is minimized.

As resistance decreases, the current dissipation also decreases. Therefore if the resistance is reduced, the energy required to maintain the magnetic field is decreased. As temperature decreases, resistance also decreases. As absolute zero of temperature (−273°C or 4°K) is approached resistance is virtually absent, so that a high magnetic field can be maintained with no input power or driving voltage required. This is the basis of the function of the supercooled, superconducting magnet. The direction of the main magnetic field runs horizontally like that of the resistive system, from the head to the feet of the magnet (Figure 51.3).

Initially, current is passed through the loops of wire to create the magnetic field or bring the field up to strength (ramping). Then the wires are supercooled with substances known as cryogens (usually liquid helium [He] or liquid nitrogen [N]), to eliminate resistance. Since He and N are stable, they can be placed into a vacuum so that they do not rapidly boil off or return to their gaseous state. This is called a **cryogen bath**, which actually surrounds the coils of wire and is housed in the system between insulated vacuums (see Figure 53.1).

Advantages

High magnetic field strengths with low power requirements are achievable. The operating costs are low. With resistance virtually eliminated, there is no longer a mechanism to dissipate current, therefore no additional power input is required to maintain the high magnetic field strength. Advanced applications and optimum image quality are possible.

Disadvantages

There are high capital costs. Fringe fields are significant, so shielding is necessary. Tunnel design renders this unsuitable for large or claustrophobic patients. Interventional and dynamic studies are difficult. However, open systems are also available (Figure 51.4).

Shim coils

Due to design limitations it is almost impossible to create an electromagnet with coils of wire that are spaced evenly (equidistant from one end of the solenoid to the other). As the strength of the field is dependent on the distance between the loops, unevenly spaced loops create sags or **inhomogeneities** in the main magnetic field. These are measured in parts per million (ppm).

To correct for these inhomogeneities, another loop of current-carrying wire is placed in the area of the inhomogeneity. This, in effect, compensates for the sag in the main magnetic field and thus creates magnetic field homogeneity or evenness. This process is called **shimming** and the extra loop of wire is called a **shim coil**. For imaging purposes, homogeneity of the order of 10 ppm is required. Spectroscopic procedures require a more homogeneous environment of 1 ppm.

The key points of this chapter are summarized in Table 51.1.

Table 51.1 Key points.
Things to remember:
Superconducting magnets are the commonest type of magnet used in clinical MRI.
The resistivity of the electromagnetic coils is zero, because they are immersed in a cryogen that reduces their temperature to absolute zero.
Current therefore flows and the magnetic field is retained as long as the electromagnetic coils have no resistance.
High magnetic strengths permit fast imaging and produces images with a good SNR. However some artefacts (e.g. chemical shift and phase mismapping) are more evident at higher field strengths.

 Access Animation 9.1 relating to this chapter at www.westbrookmriinpractice.com/animations.asp

52 Radiofrequency coils

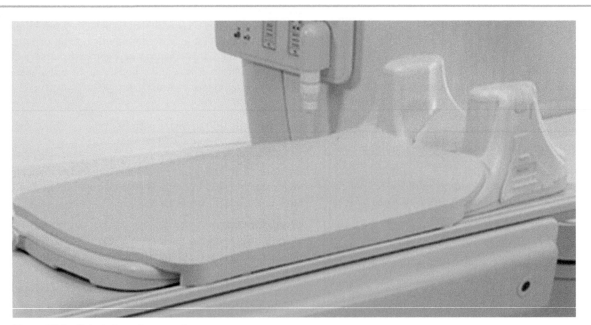

Figure 52.1 Spinal phased array coil.

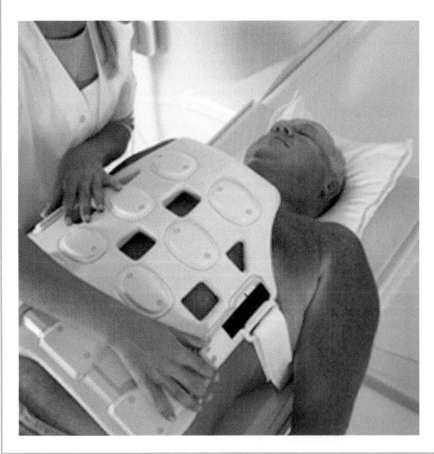

Figure 52.2 Parallel imaging coils.

MRI at a Glance, Third Edition. Catherine Westbrook. © 2016 John Wiley & Sons, Ltd. Published 2016 by John Wiley & Sons, Ltd.
Companion website: www.ataglanceseries.com/mri

RF coils consist of loops of wire that, when a current is passed through them, produce a magnetic field at 90° to B_0.

Transmit coils

Energy is transmitted at the resonant frequency of hydrogen in the form of a short, intense burst of radiofrequency known as a radiofrequency pulse. The main coils that transmit RF in most systems are:
- a body coil usually located within the bore of the magnet;
- a head coil.

The body coil is the main RF transmitter and transmits RF for most examinations, excluding head imaging (when the head coil is used). The body and head coil are also capable of receiving RF; that is, acting as receiver coils.

Receiver coils

RF coils placed in the transverse plane generate a voltage when a moving magnetic field cuts across the loops of wire. This voltage is the MR signal that is sampled to form an image. In order to induce an MR signal, the transverse magnetization must occur perpendicular to the receiver coils (see Chapter 39).

RF coil types

The configuration of the RF transmitter and receiver coils directly affects the quality of the MR signal. There are several types of coil currently used in MR imaging.

Transmit/receive coils

A coil both transmits RF and receives the MR signal and is often called a transceiver. It encompasses the entire anatomy and can be used for either head or total body imaging. Head and body coils of a type known as the birdcage configuration are used to image relatively large areas and yield uniform SNR over the entire imaging volume. However, even though the volume coils are responsible for uniform excitation over a large area, because of their great size they generally produce images with lower SNR than other types of coil. The signal quality produced by these coils is significantly increased by a process known as quadrature excitation and detection.

Surface coils

Coils of this type are used to improve the SNR when imaging structures near the surface of the patient. Generally, the nearer the coil is situated to the structure under examination, the greater the SNR. This is because the coil is closer to the signal-emitting anatomy, and only noise in the vicinity of the coil is received rather than the entire body. Surface coils are usually small and especially shaped so that they can be easily placed near the anatomy to be imaged with little or no discomfort to the patient. However, signal (and noise) is received only from the sensitive volume of the coil, which corresponds to the area located around the coil. The size of this area extends to the circumference of the coil and at a depth into the patient equal to the radius of the coil. There is therefore a fall-off of signal as the distance from the coil is increased in any direction.

Intra-cavity coils (such as rectal coils) or local coils can be used to receive signal deep within the patient. As the SNR is enhanced when using local coils, greater spatial resolution of small structures can often be achieved. When using local coils, the body coil is used to transmit RF and the local coil is used to receive the MR signal.

Phased array coils (linear array)

These consist of multiple coils and receivers whose individual signals are combined to create one image with improved SNR and increased coverage. Therefore the advantages of small surface coils (increased SNR and resolution) are combined with a large FOV for increased anatomy coverage. Usually up to four coils and receivers are grouped together, either to increase longitudinal coverage or to improve uniformity across a whole volume. During data acquisition, each individual coil receives signal from its own small, usable FOV. The signal output from each coil is separately received and processed, but then combined to form one single, larger FOV. As each coil has its own receiver, the amount of noise received is limited to its small FOV, and all the data is acquired in a single sequence rather than in four individual sequences (Figure 52.1).

Parallel imaging coils (volume array)

Parallel imaging technology has been discussed previously (see Chapter 38). This technique uses multiple coils (also known as channels) placed around the imaging volume (Figure 52.2). During each acquisition, each coil sends data to its own unique K space line so that K space is filled more rapidly. For example, if four coils or channels are used, K space may be filled four lines at a time. This technique can be used with any sequence.

Large coil
- Large area of uniform signal reception.
- Increased likelihood of aliasing (see Chapter 44).
- Positioning of patient not too critical.
- Lower SNR and resolution (see Chapters 39 and 41).

Small coil
- Small area of signal reception.
- Less likely to produce aliasing artefact.
- Positioning of coil critical.
- High SNR and resolution.

The key points of this chapter are summarized in Table 52.1.

Table 52.1 Key points.

Things to remember:
Receiver coils are a critical part of image optimization. The selection of the right coil for the area under examination is very important.
Large coils provide large coverage but a relatively poor SNR. This is because noise is received from the entire imaging volume.
Small coils provide small coverage but relatively good SNR. This is because the imaging volume is small and therefore noise is reduced.
Phase array coils of the linear and volume type are the best option, as they combine the benefits of using small coils with those of using large ones.

Access Animation 9.3 relating to this chapter at **www** **.westbrookmriinpractice.com/animations.asp**

53 Gradients and other hardware

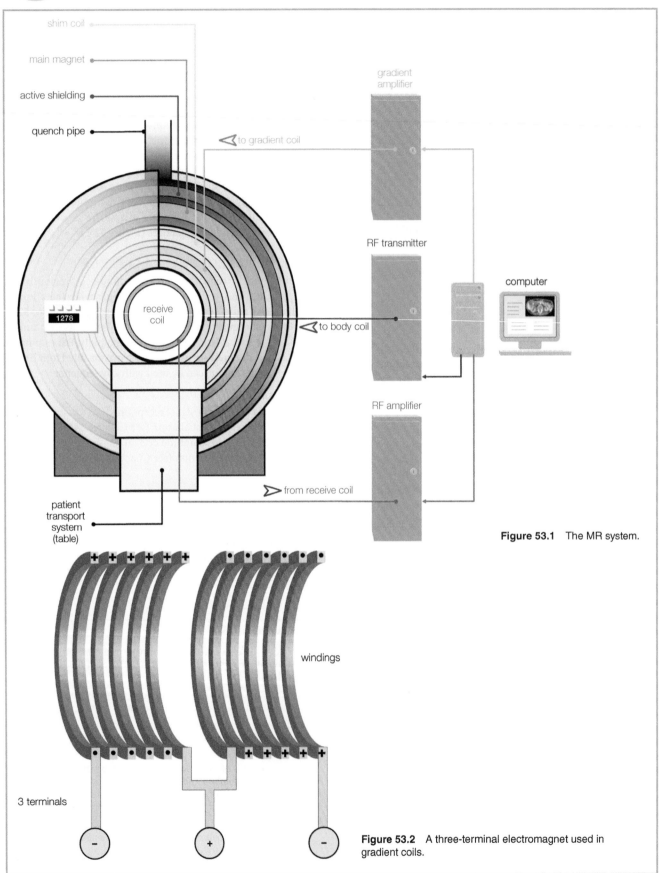

Figure 53.1 The MR system.

Figure 53.2 A three-terminal electromagnet used in gradient coils.

MRI at a Glance, Third Edition. Catherine Westbrook. © 2016 John Wiley & Sons, Ltd. Published 2016 by John Wiley & Sons, Ltd.
Companion website: www.ataglanceseries.com/mri

The components of the MR system are shown in Figure 53.1.

Gradients

Gradient coils provide a linear gradation or slope of the magnetic field strength from one end of the magnet to the other. This is achieved by passing current through the gradient coils (see Chapter 27).

The *direction* of the current through the coil determines whether the magnetic field strength is increased or decreased relative to isocentre; that is, its polarity.

The *polarity* of the current flowing through the coil determines which end of the gradient is higher than isocentre (positive) and which end is lower (negative). (See Figure 53.2.)

Gradient coils are powered by **gradient amplifiers**. There are two gradient amplifiers for each gradient, one affixed to the high end of the gradient, the other to the low. Faults in the gradients or gradient amplifiers can result in geometric distortions in the MR image.

By varying the magnetic field strength, gradients provide position-dependent variation of signal frequency and are therefore used for:
- slice selection;
- frequency encoding;
- phase encoding;
- rewinding;
- spoiling.

To apply a gradient, current is passed through a gradient coil. The change in field strength gradually increases to maximum, dependent on the magnitude of the current. The gradient remains at maximum for a specific period of time and is then switched off. The change in field strength gradually decreases until there is no change; that is, the magnetic field strength along the bore is equal to the main field strength of the magnet.

The maximum amplitude of a gradient is the maximum change of field strength per metre along the bore of the magnet that is achievable. This factor determines the maximum resolution possible because:
- steep slice select gradients are required for thin slices;
- steep phase-encoding gradients are required for fine phase matrices;
- steep frequency-encoding gradients are required for small fields of view.

The **rise time** of a gradient is the time required to achieve the maximum amplitude.

The **slew rate** is a function of rise time and amplitude. These factors determine the shortest scan times achievable.

The **duty cycle** is the percentage of time the gradient is at maximum amplitude.

The pulse control unit

The pulse control unit is responsible for synchronizing the application of the gradients and RF pulses in a pulse sequence. Gradient coils are switched on and off very rapidly and at precise times during the pulse sequence. Gradient amplifiers supply the power to the gradient coils and a pulse control unit coordinates the functions of the gradient amplifiers and the coils, so that they can be switched on and off at the appropriate times.

RF at the resonant frequency is transmitted by the RF transceiver, passes through frequency synthesizers to the RF amplifier and then through an RF monitor, which ensures that safe levels of RF are delivered to the patient. The received RF signal from the coil is filtered, amplified and digitized and then passes to the array processor for fast Fourier transform (FFT). This data is then transmitted to the image processor so that each pixel can be allocated a greyscale colour in the image.

The operator interface

MRI computer systems vary with manufacturer. Most consist of:
- a minicomputer with expansion capabilities;
- an array processor for Fourier transformation;
- an image processor that takes data from the array processor to form an image;
- hard disc drives for storage of raw data and pulse sequence parameters;
- a power distribution mechanism to distribute and filter the alternating current.

Data storage

For permanent storage of MR image data, data may be archived to an optical disc. Images are stored for viewing by a radiologist and so that cases can be retrieved for further manipulation and imaging in the future. They may also be used for comparison when repeat examinations are performed on the same patient.

The key points of this chapter are summarized in Table 53.1.

Table 53.1 Key points.
Things to remember:
There are 3 gradients, x,y and z, that perform several functions during a sequence.
The amplitude of a gradient is determined by the amount of current passing through the coil.
The polarity of a gradient is determined by the direction of the current flowing through the coil.
The amplitude of a gradient determines the spatial resolution.
The slew rate determines how fast data can be acquired.

54 # MR safety – bio-effects

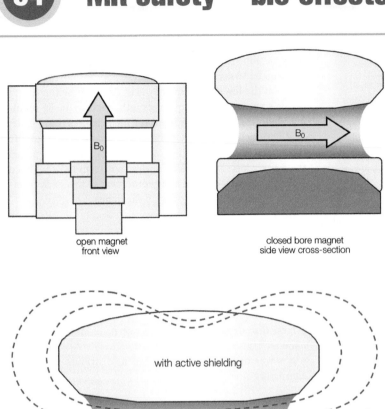

open magnet
front view

closed bore magnet
side view cross-section

Figure 54.1 Static field in permanent and superconducting systems.

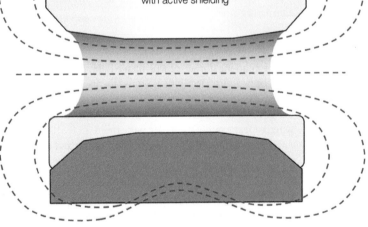

with active shielding

Figure 54.2 The fringe field.

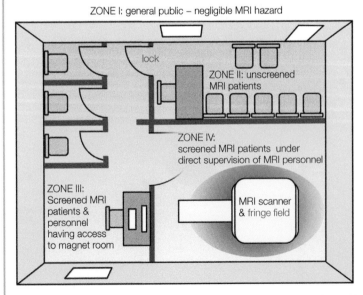

ZONE I: general public – negligible MRI hazard

lock

ZONE II: unscreened MRI patients

ZONE IV:
screened MRI patients under direct supervision of MRI personnel

ZONE III:
Screened MRI patients & personnel having access to magnet room

MRI scanner & fringe field

Figure 54.3 The zoning recommended by the American College of Radiology White Paper on MRI safety. Note that there has to be locked access between Zones II and III.

MRI at a Glance, Third Edition. Catherine Westbrook. © 2016 John Wiley & Sons, Ltd. Published 2016 by John Wiley & Sons, Ltd.

Companion website: www.ataglanceseries.com/mri

Static magnetic field bio-effects

Current guidelines recommend a maximum limit of 8 T for clinical imaging, rising to 12 T for research purposes and spectroscopy. Most clinical units operate below 3 T.

The following points are *fundamentally* important with regard to the potentially harmful effects of the static magnetic field. The static field is always present (24 hours a day, 365 days a year, to infinity). It is switched on even when the system is out of use (Figure 54.1). The fringe field may extend several metres beyond the examination room and therefore any harmful effects or risks may come into play at some distance from the scanner (Figure 54.2).

There is no conclusive evidence for irreversible or harmful bio-effects in humans below 2.5 T. Reversible abnormalities may include:
- an increase in the amplitude of the T-wave that can be noted on an ECG due to the magnetic hydrodynamic effect (also known as the magnetic haemodynamic effect);
- heating of patients;
- fatigue;
- headaches;
- hypotension;
- irritability.

Time-varying field bio-effects

Gradients create a time-varying magnetic field. This changing field occurs during the scanning sequence. It is not present at other times and therefore exposure is restricted to patients and to relatives who may be present in the scan room during the examination (see Scan Tips 14 and 15).

The health consequences are not related to the strength of the gradient field, but to changes in the magnetic field that cause induced currents. Nerves, blood vessels and muscles, which act as conductors in the body, may be affected. The induced current is greater in peripheral tissues, since the amplitude of the gradient is higher away from magnetic isocentre.

Time-varying bio-effects from gradient coils include:
- light flashes in the eyes;
- alterations in the biochemistry of cells and fracture union;
- mild cutaneous sensations;
- involuntary muscle contractions;
- cardiac arrhythmias.

RF transmit coils also produce time-varying fields. The predominant bio-effect of RF irradiation absorption is the potential heating of tissue. As an excitation pulse is applied, some nuclei absorb the RF energy and enter the high-energy state. As they relax, nuclei give off this absorbed energy to the surrounding lattice. As excitation frequency is increased, absorbed energy is also increased, therefore heating of tissue is largely frequency dependent.

Energy dissipation can be described in terms of **specific absorption rate** or **SAR**. SAR is expressed in watts per kilogram (W/kg), a quantity that depends on:
- induced electrical field;
- pulse duty cycle;
- tissue density;
- conductivity;
- the size of the patient.

SAR is used to calculate an expected increase in body temperature during an average examination (Table 54.1). In the UK, it is recommended that this should not exceed 1° C during the examination. Studies show that patient exposure up to three times the recommended levels produces no serious adverse effects, despite elevations in skin and body temperatures. As body temperature increases, blood pressure and heart rate also increase slightly. Even though these effects seem insignificant, patients with compromised thermoregulatory systems may not be candidates for MRI.

Table 54.1 SAR limits in the USA.

Area	Dose	Time (mins)	SAR (W/kg)
Whole body	averaged over	15	4
Head	averaged over	10	3
Head or torso	per gram of tissue	5	8
Extremities	per gram of tissue	5	12

Radiofrequency fields can be responsible for significant burn hazards due to electrical currents that are produced in conductive loops. Equipment used in MRI, such as ECG leads and surface coils, should therefore be employed with extreme caution. When using a surface coil, the operator must be careful to prevent any electrically conductive material (e.g. cable of surface coil) from forming a 'conductive loop' with itself or with the patient.

Site planning

There have been a number of fatal accidents in the MR environment. It is therefore vital that access to the MRI system and the magnetic field is controlled. The American College of Radiologists has produced a White Paper that recommends that all centres define the following zones (Figure 54.3).

Zone I includes all areas that are accessible to the public. All personnel are allowed in Zone I.

Zone II is the interface between Zone I and the controlled Zone III. There must be a lock or warning signs between Zones I and II. All personnel are allowed in Zone II, but there should be a trained 'gate-keeper' to keep patients and non-MR personnel from inadvertently entering Zones II and IV.

Zone III is strictly restricted because free access by unscreened personnel and ferromagnetic objects may cause death or serious injury. This area must be strictly monitored and only MR-trained personnel and screened patients are permitted in this area.

Zone IV is only suitable for screened patients under direct and constant supervision from MR-trained personnel, as death and serious injury can occur. The patient may also experience heating, missile effects, RF antenna effects and anoxia in this zone.

The key points of this chapter are summarized in Table 54.2.

Table 54.2 Key points.

Things to remember:
The magnetic field is present 24 hours a day, 365 days of the year.
There is no conclusive evidence that the static magnetic field is harmful up to 2.5T.
Time-varying fields imposed by the gradients can have effects, especially when using very fast sequences.
RF pulses can cause heating. The SAR is a measure of how much energy the patient's tissues absorb during the scan.
Site planning requires the establishment of clearly marked zones.

Access Scan Tips 14 and 15 and the MCQs relating to this chapter on the book's companion website at www.ataglanceseries.com/mri

Access Animation 9.2 relating to this chapter at www.westbrookmriinpractice.com/animations.asp

55 MR safety – projectiles

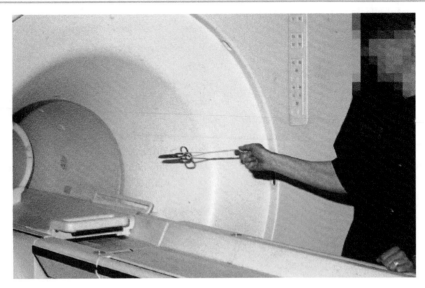

Figure 55.1 The pulling power of a pair of scissors in a 1.5 T system.

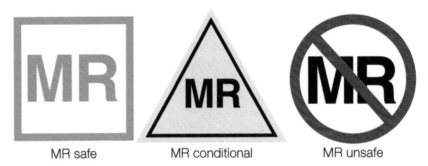

MR safe   MR conditional   MR unsafe

Figure 55.2 Standard labels associated with MR device testing.

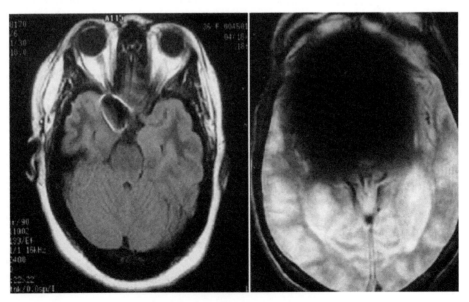

Figure 55.3 Patient with an intracranial vascular clip using spin echo (left) and gradient echo MRI (right). Magnetic susceptibility artefact is clearly seen on the gradient echo image.

MRI at a Glance, Third Edition. Catherine Westbrook. © 2016 John Wiley & Sons, Ltd. Published 2016 by John Wiley & Sons, Ltd.
Companion website: www.ataglanceseries.com/mri

The projectile effect of a metal object exposed to the field can seriously compromise the safety of anyone sited between the object and the magnet system. *The potential harm cannot be over-emphasized.* In many ways the MR scan room is the most dangerous room in a hospital or imaging facility, because it is possible to seriously injure or even kill someone in a second. Even small objects such as paperclips and hairpins have a terminal velocity of 40 mph when pulled into a 1.5 T magnet, and therefore pose a serious risk to the patient and anyone else present in the scan room. Larger objects such as scissors travel at much higher velocities and may be fatal to any person in their path (Figure 55.1).

Many types of clinical equipment are ferromagnetic and should **never** be brought into the scan room. These include surgical tools, scissors, clamps and oxygen tanks (see Scan Tips 14 and 15).

Quenching

If an accident occurs where a patient or other person in the scan room is pinned to the magnet by a projectile that cannot be removed by hand, the magnetic field must be immediately quenched. Quenching is the process whereby there is a sudden loss of absolute zero of temperature in the magnet coils, so that they cease to be superconducting and become resistive. The magnetic field is therefore lost. Quenching can be initiated on purpose, usually by pressing a quench button in the control room, or it may happen accidently. Quenching causes helium to escape from the cryogen bath extremely rapidly. Quenching may cause severe and irreparable damage to the superconducting coils, and so all systems should have helium-venting equipment, which removes the helium to the outside environment in the event of a quench. However, if this fails, helium vents into the room and replaces oxygen. For this reason, all scan rooms should contain an oxygen monitor that sounds an alarm if the oxygen falls below a certain level.

Metallic implants and prostheses

Devices are tested on an ongoing basis for MR safety and many manufacturers have developed MR-safe devices. It is therefore vital to check the type of device or implant and whether it is safe before booking the appointment. Metallic implants and prostheses produce serious effects, which include torque or twisting in the field, heating effects and artefacts on MR images. The type of metal used in such implants is one factor that determines the force exerted on them in magnetic fields. While non-ferrous metallic implants may show little or no deflection to the field, they could cause significant heating due to their inability to dissipate the heat caused by radiofrequency absorption. Devices that might need to be taken into the scan room must be tested beforehand. There are standard labels depending on whether the device is safe, unsafe or conditional on the field strength (Figure 55.2).

What is not safe to scan?

Cochlear implants are attracted to the magnetic field and are magnetically or electronically activated. They are therefore unsafe to scan.

It is not uncommon for patients who have worked with sheet metal to have metal fragments or slivers located in and around the eye. Since the magnetic field exerts a force on ferromagnetic objects, a metal fragment in the eye could move or be displaced and cause injury to the eye or surrounding tissue. Therefore all patients with a suspected eye injury must be X-rayed before the MR examination.

Aneurysm clip motion may damage the vessel, resulting in haemorrhage, ischaemia or death. Currently, many intracranial clips are made of a non-ferromagnetic substance such as titanium. However, some of these may still deflect in a magnetic field. It is therefore recommended that imaging of patients with aneurysm clips is delayed, until the type of clip is emphatically identified as non-ferrous and non-deflectable. Intracranial clips also cause severe magnetic susceptibility artefact, especially in gradient echo sequences (Figure 55.3).

Although MR-safe pacemakers have been developed, it is important to assume that most patients do not have this kind of pacemaker. Even field strengths as low as 10 gauss may be sufficient to cause deflection, programming changes and closure of the reed switch that converts a pacemaker to asynchronous mode. Patients who have had their pacemaker removed may have pacer wires left within the body that could act as an antenna and (by induced currents) cause cardiac fibrillation.

What is probably safe to scan?

Prosthetic heart valves are deflected by the static magnetic field, but this is minimal compared to normal pulsatile cardiac motion. Although patients with most valvular implants are considered safe for MR, careful screening for valve type is advised.

Most orthopaedic implants show no deflection within the main magnetic field. A large metallic implant such as a hip prosthesis can become heated by currents induced in the metal by the magnetic and radiofrequency fields. It appears, however, that such heating is relatively low. The majority of orthopaedic implants have been imaged with MR without incident.

Abdominal surgical clips are generally safe for MR because they become anchored by fibrous tissue, but produce artefacts in proportion to their size and can distort the image.

The key points of this chapter are summarized in Table 55.1.

Table 55.1 Key points.
Things to remember:
The MR scan room can be considered the most dangerous room in the hospital or imaging facility.
Objects are accelerated towards the magnet at very high velocity depending on their mass, the strength of the magnetic field and what they are made of.
Anyone entering the scan room must have been thoroughly screened and checked by a trained MR practitioner.
Implants and any devices being taken into the scan room must be checked beforehand.

 Access Scan Tips 14 and 15 and the MCQs relating to this chapter on the book's companion website at www.ataglanceseries.com/mri

Appendix 1(a): The results of optimizing image quality

To optimize image	Adjusted parameter	Trade-off
Maximize SNR	↑ NSA	↑ scan time ↓ motion artefact
	↓ phase matrix	↓ scan time ↓ spatial resolution
	↑ slice thickness	↓ spatial resolution
	↓ receive bandwidth	↑ minimum TE ↑ chemical shift
	↑ FOV	↓ spatial resolution
	↑ TR	↓ T1 weighting (TR < 2000 ms) ↑ number of slices
	↓ TE	↓ T2 weighting
Maximize spatial resolution (assuming a square FOV)	↓ slice thickness	↓ SNR
	↑ matrix	↓ SNR ↑ scan time (phase matrix)
	↓ FOV	↓ SNR
Minimize scan time	↓ TR	↑ T1 weighting (TR < 2000 ms) ↓ SNR (TR < 2000 ms) ↓ number of slices
	↓ phase matrix	↓ spatial resolution ↑ SNR
	↓ NSA	↓ SNR ↑ movement artefact
	↓ slice number in volume imaging	↓ SNR and coverage

Appendix 1(b): Parameters and their associated trade-offs

Parameter	Benefit	Limitation
TR increased	increased SNR increased number of slices	increased scan time decreased T1 weighting
TR decreased	decreased scan time increased T1 weighting	decreased SNR decreased number of slices
TE increased	increased T2 weighting	decreased SNR
TE decreased	increased SNR	decreased T2 weighting
NEX increased	increased SNR more signal averaging	direct proportional increase in scan time
NEX decreased	direct proportional decrease in scan time	decreased SNR less signal averaging
Slice thickness increased	increased SNR increased coverage of anatomy	decreased spatial resolution more partial voluming
Slice thickness decreased	increased spatial resolution reduced partial voluming	decreased SNR decreased coverage of anatomy
FOV increased	increased SNR increased coverage of anatomy	decreased spatial resolution decreased likelihood of aliasing
FOV decreased	increased spatial resolution increased likelihood of aliasing	decreased SNR decreased coverage of anatomy
Matrix increased	increased spatial resolution	increased scan time (phase matrix) decreased SNR if voxel is small
Matrix decreased	decreased scan time (phase matrix) increased SNR if voxel is large	decreased spatial resolution
Receive bandwidth increased	decrease in chemical shift decrease in minimum TE	decreased SNR
Receive bandwidth decreased	increased SNR	increase in chemical shift increase in minimum TE
Large coil	increased area of received signal	lower SNR aliasing with small FOV
Small coil	increased SNR less prone to aliasing with a small FOV	decreased area of received signal

Appendix 2: Artefacts and their remedies

Artefact	Axis	Remedy	Penalty
Truncation	phase	increase number of K space lines filled with data (increase phase matrix and do not use partial Fourier techniques)	increase scan time
Flow	phase	pre-saturation pulses	may lose a slice increase SAR
		gradient moment rephasing	increase minimum TE
Chemical shift	frequency	increase receive bandwidth	decrease minimum TE decrease SNR
		reduce FOV	reduce SNR
		use chemical saturation	reduce SNR
Out-of-phase artefact	frequency and phase	select a TE at periodicity of fat and water	may lose a slice if TE is significantly reduced
Aliasing		no phase wrap	may increase scan time depending on manufacturer
		enlarge phase FOV	increase scan time reduce resolution
Zipper	frequency	call engineer	irate engineer!
Magnetic susceptibility	frequency and phase	use spin echo sequences	Cannot use gradient echo sequences unless specifically wishing to enhance susceptibility
		remove metal	none
Shading	frequency and phase	check shim	none
		load coil correctly	none
Motion	phase	use anti-spasmodics	costly invasive
		immobilize patient	none
		counselling of patient	none
		sedation	possible side effects invasive costly requires monitoring
		respiratory compensation or breath-holding techniques	scan time may increase
		cardiac or peripheral gating	scan time increases
		pre-saturation pulses	increase SAR may reduce slice number
Cross-talk	slice select	interleaving	doubles the scan time
		squaring off RF pulses	reduce SNR
		large slice gap	fewer slices and missed anatomy
Moiré	frequency and phase	use spin echo sequences	none
		patient not to touch bore	none
Magic angle	frequency	change TE	none
		alter position of anatomy	none

Appendix 3: Main manufacturers' acronyms

	GE	Philips	Siemens
Spin echo	SE	SE	SE
Fast spin echo	FSE	TSE	TSE
Inversion recovery	IR	IR	IR
Short tau inversion recovery	STIR	STIR	STIR
Fluid attenuated inversion recovery	FLAIR	FLAIR	FLAIR
Coherent gradient echo	GRASS	FFE	FISP
Incoherent gradient echo	SPGR	T1 FFE	FLASH
Balanced gradient echo	FIESTA	BFFE	True FISP
Steady-state free precession	SSFP	T2 FFE	PSIF
Fast gradient echo	Fast GRASS/SPGR	TFE	Turbo FLASH
Echo planar	EPI	EPI	EPI
Parallel imaging	ASSET	SENSE	iPAT
Spatial pre-saturation	SAT	REST	SAT
Gradient moment rephasing	Flow comp	Flow comp	GMR
Signal averaging	NEX	NSA	NSA
Anti-aliasing	No phase wrap	Fold-over suppression	Phase oversampling
Rectangular FOV	Rect FOV	Rect FOV	Half Fourier imaging
Respiratory compensation	Resp comp	PEAR	Resp trigger

Abbreviations used above

ASSET	array spatial and sensitivity encoding technique
FFE	fast field echo
FIESTA	free induction echo stimulated acquisition
FISP	free induction steady precession
FLAIR	fluid attenuated inversion recovery
FLASH	fast low-angled shot
Flow comp	flow compensation
FSE	fast spin echo
GMR	gradient moment rephasing
GRASS	gradient recalled acquisition in the steady state
iPAT	integrated parallel acquisition technique
MP RAGE	magnetization prepared rapid gradient echo
NEX	number of excitations
NSA	number of signal averages
PEAR	phase-encoding artefact reduction
PSIF	mirrored FISP
REST	regional saturation technique
SENSE	sensitivity encoding
SPGR	spoiled GRASS
SSFP	steady-state free precession
STIR	short tau inversion recovery
TFE	turbo field echo
TSE	turbo spin echo
Turbo FLASH	magnetization prepared sub-second imaging

Glossary

2D volumetric acquisition acquisition where a small amount of data is acquired from each slice before repeating the TR

3D volumetric acquisition acquisition where the whole imaging volume is excited so that the images can be viewed in any plane

Actual TE the time between the echo and the next RF pulse in SSFP

Aliasing artefact produced when anatomy outside the FOV is mismapped inside the FOV

Alignment when nuclei are placed in an external magnetic field their magnetic moments line up with the magnetic field flux lines

Alnico alloy that is used to make permanent magnets

Ampere's law determines the magnitude and direction of the magnetic field due to a current; if you point your right thumb along the direction of the current, then the magnetic field points along the direction of the curled fingers

Analogue to digital conversion (ADC) process by which a waveform is sampled and digitized

Angular momentum the spin of MR active nuclei that depends on the balance between the number of protons and neutrons in the nucleus

Anti-parallel alignment describes the alignment of magnetic moments in the opposite direction to the main field

Apparent diffusion coefficient (ADC) net displacement of molecules due to diffusion

Atomic number sum of protons in the nucleus

B_0 the main magnetic field measured in tesla

b value strength and duration of diffusion gradients

Balanced gradient echo (BGE) gradient echo sequence that uses balanced gradients and alternating RF pulses

Bipolar describes a magnet with two poles, north and south

Blipping where the phase-encoding gradient slope is slighted altered to jump from one K space line to the next

Blood oxygen level dependent (BOLD) a functional MRI technique that utilizes the differences in magnetic susceptibility between oxyhaemoglobin and deoxyhaemoglobin to image areas of activated cerebral cortex

Brownian motion internal motion of the molecules

Cardiac gating monitors cardiac electrical activity during the sequence to reduce cardiac wall motion artefact

Centric K space filling Central lines area of K space filled with the shallowest phase-encoding slopes first and outer lines later

Cerebral blood volume (CBV) volume of blood perfusing through the brain per unit time

Chemical shift the precessional frequency difference between fat and water

Chemical shift artefact along the frequency axis caused by the frequency difference between fat and water

Classical theory uses the direction of the magnetic moments to illustrate alignment

Co-current flow flow in the same direction as slice excitation

Coherent the magnetic moments of hydrogen are at the same place on the precessional path

Coherent gradient echo (CGE) gradient echo sequence that uses rewinder gradients

Conjugate symmetry symmetry of data in K space

Contrast to noise ratio (CNR) difference in SNR between two adjacent structures

Countercurrent flow flow in the opposite direction to slice excitation

Cross-talk energy given to nuclei in adjacent slices by the RF pulse

Cryogen bath area around the coils of wire in which cryogens are placed

Cryogens substances used to supercool the coils of wire in a superconducting magnet

Data point digitized data that contains spatial frequency information as a result of spatial encoding

Decay loss of coherent transverse magnetization

Dephasing the magnetic moments of hydrogen are at a different place on their precessional path

Diamagnetism property that shows a small magnetic moment that opposes the applied field

Diffusion a term used to describe moving molecules due to random thermal motion

Diffusion tensor imaging (DTI) DWI sequence that uses very strong multidirectional gradients

Diffusion weighted imaging (DWI) sequence that uses gradients to sensitize the sequence to diffusion

Dipole-dipole interaction the phenomenon by which excited protons are affected by nearby excited protons and electrons

Dixon technique technique that uses a TE when fat and water are out of phase with each other to null the signal from fat

Drive see Fast recovery

Driven equilibrium a sequence that uses additional pulses to drive any remaining transverse magnetization into the longitudinal plane

Duty cycle the percentage of time a gradient is at maximum amplitude

Echo planar imaging (EPI) sequence that uses single and multi-shot K space filling techniques with sampling of gradient echoes

Echo spacing spacing between each echo in TSE

Echo train series of 180° rephasing pulse and echoes in a turbo spin echo pulse sequence

Echo train length (ETL) the number of 180° RF pulses and resultant echoes in TSE

Effective TE the time between the echo and the RF pulse that initiated it in SSFP and TSE sequences

Electrons orbit the nucleus in distinct shells and are negatively charged

emf drives a current in a circuit and is the result of a changing magnetic field inducing an electric field

Entry slice phenomena contrast difference of flowing nuclei relative to the stationary nuclei because they are fresh

Ernst angle the flip angle that results in the highest signal intensity in a tissue with a particular T1 relaxation time and at a particular TR

Excitation the energy transfer from the RF pulse to the spins

Extrinsic contrast parameters contrast parameters that are controlled by the system operator

Faraday's law of induction law that states that a change of magnetic flux induces an emf in a closed circuit

Fast Fourier transform (FFT) mathematical conversion of frequency/time domain to frequency/amplitude

Fast recovery FSE sequence that uses an additional RF pulse to drive any residual transverse magnetization into the longitudinal plane (also called Drive)

Fast spin echo (FSE) spin echo sequence that decreases scan time by filling multiple lines of K space every TR (also called turbo spin echo)

Ferromagnetism property of a substance that ensures that it remains magnetic, is permanently magnetized and subsequently becomes a permanent magnet

Field of view (FOV) area of anatomy covered in an image

FLAIR (fluid attenuated inversion recovery) IR sequences that nulls the signal from CSF

Fleming's right-hand rule see Ampere's law

Flip angle the angle of the NMV to B_0

Flow compensation see Gradient moment nulling

Flow-encoding axes axes along which bipolar gradients act in order to sensitize flow along the axis of the gradient; used in phase contrast MRA

Flow phenomena artefacts produced by flowing nuclei

Flow-related enhancement decrease in time of flight due to a decrease in velocity of flow

Free induction decay (FID) loss of signal due to relaxation

Frequency the speed with which a spin precesses or a waveform oscillates

Frequency encoding locating a signal according to its frequency

Frequency matrix number of pixels in the frequency direction of an image

Frequency shift difference in frequency between spins located along a gradient

Fresh spins nuclei that have not been beaten down by repeated RF pulses

Fringe field stray magnetic field outside the bore of the magnet

Functional MR imaging (fMRI) a rapid MR imaging technique that acquires images of the brain during activity or stimulus and at rest

Gadolinium (Gd) positive contrast agent

Gauss (G) unit of field strength; 1 tesla = 10,000 gauss

Ghosting motion artefact in the phase axis

Gradient amplifier supplies power to the gradient coils

Gradient echo (GE) echo produced as a result of gradient rephasing

Gradient echo pulse sequence one that uses a gradient to regenerate an echo

Gradient moment nulling (GMN) uses additional gradients to reduce flow artefact

Gradient spoiling the use of gradients to dephase magnetic moments; the opposite of rewinding

Gradients coils of wire that alter the magnetic field strength in a linear fashion when a current is passed through them

Gyromagnetic ratio the precessional frequency of an element at 1 T

High-velocity signal loss increase in time of flight due to an increase in the velocity of flow

Homogeneity the evenness of the magnetic field

Hybrid sequences sequences where a series of gradient echoes are interspersed with 180° rephasing pulses; in this way susceptibility artefacts are reduced

Hyperintense high signal intensity (bright)

Hypointense low signal intensity (dark)

Image matrix a grid of matrix of pixels that divide up the FOV

Incoherent means that the magnetic moments of hydrogen are at different places on the precessional path

Incoherent gradient echo gradient echo sequence that uses RF spoiling for T1 weighting

Induced electric current oscillating current that occurs when a magnet is moved in a closed circuit

Inflow effect another term for entry slice phenomenon

Inhomogeneities areas where the magnetic field strength is not exactly the same as the main field strength

Intra-voxel dephasing phase difference between flow and stationary nuclei in a voxel

Intrinsic contrast mechanisms contrast parameters that do not come under the operator's control

Inversion recovery (IR) sequence that uses an inverting pulse to saturate or null tissue

Ions atoms with an excess or deficit of electrons

Isointense same signal intensity

Isotopes atoms of the same element having a different mass number

J coupling a process that describes the reduction the spin-spin interactions cause in fat, thereby increasing its T2 decay time

Kilogauss (kG) unit of field strength (1000 gauss)

K space an area where raw data is stored

Larmor equation used to calculate the frequency or speed of precession for a specific nucleus in a specific magnetic field strength

Lenz's law states that induced emf is in a direction so that it opposes the change in magnetic field that causes it

Longitudinal plane the axis parallel to B_0

Magnetic flux density number of flux lines per unit area

Magnetic isocentre the centre of the bore of the magnet in all planes

Magnetic lines of flux lines of force running from the magnetic south to the north poles of the magnet

Magnetic moment denotes the direction of the north/south axis of a magnet and the amplitude of the magnetic field

Magnetic susceptibility ability of a substance to become magnetized

Magnetism a property of all matter that depends on the magnetic susceptibility of the atom

Magnetization prepared a prepulse applied before the main sequence to null the signal from certain tissues in fast gradient echo

Magnetization transfer transfer of RF energy from free to bound protons

Magnitude image unsubtracted image combination of flow-sensitized data

Mass number sum of neutrons and protons in the nucleus

Mean transit time (MTT) used in perfusion imaging to indicate the transit time of blood through a tissue

MR active nuclei that possess an odd number of protons

MR angiography method of visualizing vessels that contain flowing nuclei by producing a contrast between them and the stationary nuclei

MR signal the voltage induced in the receiver coil

Multishot (MS) technique that fills K space in multiple sections

Net magnetization vector (NMV) the magnetic vector produced as a result of the alignment of excess hydrogen nuclei with B_0

Neutrons particles in the nucleus that have no charge

Null point point at which there is no longitudinal magnetization in a tissue

Number of excitations (NEX) see Number of signal averages

Number of signal averages (NSA) the number of times each line is filled with data (also known as NEX)

Nyquist theorem states that frequencies must be sampled at a rate at least twice that of the highest frequency in the echo in order to reliably reproduce it

Off resonant RF pulses applied at a frequency slightly different to the Larmor frequency of a tissue

On resonant RF pulses applied at the Larmor frequency of a particular tissue

Outer lines area of K space filled with the steepest phase-encoding gradient slopes

Out-of-phase artefact artefact along the phase axis caused by the phase difference between fat and water

Parallel alignment describes the alignment of magnetic moments in the same direction as the main field

Parallel imaging technique that uses multiple coils to fill multiple lines of K space every TR

Paramagnetism property whereby substances affect external magnetic fields in a positive way, resulting in a local increase in the magnetic field

Partial averaging filling only a proportion of K space with data and putting zeroes in the remainder

Partial echo sampling only part of the echo and extrapolating the remainder in K space

Perfusion a measure of the quality of vascular supply to a tissue

Periodicity the time interval between the magnetic moments of fat and water being in phase

Permanent magnets magnets that retain their magnetism

Phase the position of a magnetic moment on its precessional path at any given time

Phase contrast angiography technique that generates vascular contrast by applying a bipolar gradient to different stationary and moving spins by their phase

Phase curve a waveform derived from plotting different phase positions over a distance in the patient

Phase encoding locating a signal according to its phase

Phase image subtracted image combination of flow-sensitized data

Phase matrix number of pixels in the phase direction of an image

Phase reordering the order that lines of K space are filled is altered from linear to non-linear

Phase shift difference in phase between spins located along a gradient

Pixel picture element in the FOV

Polarity the direction of a gradient, i.e. which end is greater than B_0 and which is lower than B_0; depends on the direction of the current through the gradient coil

Precession the secondary spin of magnetic moments around B_0

Precessional frequency frequency with which MR active nuclei precess when exposed to an external magnetic field

Presaturation technique that uses RF pulses before the sequence to null the signal from moving spins or from certain types of tissue

Protium isotope of hydrogen that has a mass and atomic number of 1; MR active nucleus used in MRI

Proton density the number of protons in a unit volume of tissue

Proton density weighting image that demonstrates the differences in the proton densities of the tissues

Protons particles in the nucleus that are positively charged

Pseudo-frequency the frequency derived from a waveform that represents the change of phase of spins within a voxel across the whole acquisition

Pulse control unit coordinates the switching on and off of the gradient and RF transmitter coils at appropriate times during the pulse sequence

Pulse sequence a series of RF pulses, gradient applications and intervening time periods; used to control contrast

Quantum theory uses the energy level of the nuclei to illustrate alignment

Quenching process by which there is a sudden loss of the superconductivity of the magnet coils so that the magnet becomes resistive

Radians/cm the units of K space

Radiowaves waves of electromagnetic radiation that oscillate with a radiofrequency

Ramp sampling where sampling data points are collected when the gradient rise time is almost complete; sampling occurs while the gradient is still reaching maximum amplitude, while the gradient is at maximum amplitude, and as it begins to decline

Readout gradient the frequency-encoding gradient

Receive bandwidth range of frequencies that are sampled during readout; determines the sampling rate

Recovery growth of longitudinal magnetization

Rectangular FOV FOV where the phase FOV is smaller than the frequency FOV

Relaxation process by which the NMV loses energy

Relaxivity process by which relaxation rates of a tissue are altered by administering contrast agents

Repetition time (TR) time between each excitation pulse

Rephasing creating in-phase magnetization, usually by using an RF pulse or a gradient

Residual magnetization transverse magnetization left over from previous RF pulses in steady-state conditions

Resistive magnet an electromagnet created by passing current through loops of wire

Resonance an energy transition that occurs when an object is subjected to a frequency the same as its own

Respiratory compensation uses bellows around the patient's chest to reduce respiratory motion artefact

Respiratory triggering the scan is initiated when the patient is not breathing

Rewinding the use of a gradient to rephase magnetic moments

RF amplifier supplies power to the RF transmitter coils

RF pulse short burst of RF energy that excites nuclei into a high-energy state

RF spoiling the use of digitized RF to transmit and receive at a certain phase

RF transmitter coil coil that transmits RF at the resonant frequency of hydrogen to excite nuclei and move them into a high-energy state

Rise time the time it takes a gradient to switch on, achieve the required gradient slope, and switch off again

Rotating frame of reference where you, the observer, ride along with the object that is moving

Sampling rate rate at which samples are taken during readout

Sampling time the time for which the readout gradient is switched on

Saturation occurs when the NMV is flipped to a full 180°

Sequential acquisition acquisition where all the data from each slice is acquired before going on to the next

Shim coil extra coils used to make the magnetic field as homogeneous as possible

Shimming process whereby the evenness of the magnetic field is optimized

Signal to noise ratio (SNR) ratio of signal relative to noise

Single shot (SS) a sequence where all the lines of K space are acquired at once

Slew rate function of gradient rise time and amplitude

Slice encoding the separation of individual slice locations by phase in volume acquisitions

Slice selection selecting a slice using a gradient

Spatial encoding spatially locating a signal in three dimensions

Spatial resolution the ability to distinguish two points as separate

Specific absorption rate (SAR) rate/kg at which energy from the RF pulse is dissipated

Spectroscopy provides a frequency spectrum of a given tissue based on the molecular and chemical structures of that tissue

Spin down the population of high-energy hydrogen nuclei that align their magnetic moments anti-parallel to the main field

Spin echo (SE) echo produced as a result of a 180° rephasing pulse

Spin echo pulse sequence one that uses a 180° rephasing pulse to generate an echo

Spin lattice relaxation process by which energy is given up to the surrounding lattice

Spin-spin relaxation process by which interactions between the magnetic fields of adjacent nuclei cause dephasing

Spin up the population of low-energy hydrogen nuclei that align their magnetic moments parallel to B_0

Spoiling a process of dephasing spins either with a gradient or an RF pulse

Stationary frame of reference is where you, the observer, are viewing something that is moving

Steady state a situation when the TR is shorter than both the T1 and T2 relaxation times of all the tissues

Steady-state free precession (SSFP) gradient echo sequence that uses echo shifting for T2 weighting

Stejskal Tanner scheme two gradients of equal polarity and amplitude are applied on each side of a 180° RF pulse

Stimulated echo echo produced by previous RF pulse in a steady-state sequence by rephasing residual transverse magnetization

Stimulated echo acquisition mode (STEAM) technique used in spectroscopy

STIR (short TI inversion recovery) sequence used to suppress fat

Superconducting magnet electromagnet that uses supercooled coils of wire so that there is no inherent resistance in the system; the current flows, and therefore the magnetism is generated without a driving voltage

T1 enhancement agent a paramagnetic contrast agent, e.g. gadolinium

T1 recovery growth of longitudinal magnetization as a result of spin lattice relaxation

T1 recovery time time taken for 63% of the longitudinal magnetization to recover

T1 weighted image image that demonstrates the differences in the T1 times of the tissues

T2 decay loss of coherent transverse magnetization as a result of spin-spin relaxation

T2 decay time time taken for 63% of the transverse magnetization to decay

T2 enhancement agent a super paramagnetic contrast agent, e.g. iron oxide

T2 weighted image image that demonstrates the differences in the T2 times of the tissues

T2* dephasing due to inhomogeneities

Time from inversion (TI) time between inversion and excitation in IR sequences

Tesla (T) unit of field strength

Time intensity curve used in perfusion imaging to measure perfusion kinetics of a volume of tissue

Time-of-flight angiography (TOF MRA) technique that generates vascular contrast by utilizing the inflow effect

Time-of-flight flow phenomenon rate of flow in a given time; causes some flowing nuclei to receive one RF pulse only and therefore produce a signal void

Time to echo (TE) time between the excitation pulse and the echo

Transceiver coil that both transmits RF and receives the MR signal

Transmit bandwidth range of frequencies transmitted in an RF pulse

Transverse plane the axis perpendicular to B_0

Turbo factor or echo train length the number of 180° rephasing pulse/echoes/phase encodings per TR in fast spin echo

Turbo spin echo (TSE) see Fast spin echo

Velocity encoding (VENC) sensitizes the sequence to blood flow in PC MRA

Volume coil coil that transmits and receives signal over a large volume of the patient

Voxel volume of tissue in the patient

Voxel volume size of a voxel

Watergram TSE sequence using very long TRs, TEs and turbo factors to produce very heavy T2 weighting

Weighting process by which parameters are manipulated so that one intrinsic contrast mechanism is more dominant than the others

Index

Note: Page numbers in *italics* refer to figures, those in **bold** refer to tables.

MRI at a Glance, Third Edition. Catherine Westbrook. © 2016 John Wiley & Sons, Ltd. Published 2016 by John Wiley & Sons, Ltd.
Companion website: www.ataglanceseries.com/mri